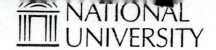

NATIONAL UNIVERSITY

LAX LIBRARY
9920 South La Cienega Blvd.
Inglewood, CA 90301
(310) 258 - 6780

Date: 5-8-00

Send book to:
San Diego

For: Student / Faculty / Staff

Name: Shamis Alshamsi

I.D. #: 3404027

Phone No.:

Staff initials: 6/11/00

Due Date:

Please do not remove the
band from this book.

Adult Development

CRITICAL ISSUES IN PSYCHIATRY
An Educational Series for Residents and Clinicians

Series Editor: Sherwyn M. Woods, M.D., Ph.D.
                   University of Southern California School of Medicine
                   Los Angeles, California

A RESIDENT'S GUIDE TO PSYCHIATRIC EDUCATION
Edited by Michael G. G. Thompson, M.D.

STATES OF MIND: Analysis of Change in Psychotherapy
Mardi J. Horowitz, M.D.

DRUG AND ALCOHOL ABUSE: A Clinical Guide to
Diagnosis and Treatment
Marc A. Schuckit, M.D.

THE INTERFACE BETWEEN THE PSYCHODYNAMIC AND
BEHAVIORAL THERAPIES
Edited by Judd Marmor, M.D., and Sherwyn M. Woods, M.D., Ph.D.

LAW IN THE PRACTICE OF PSYCHIATRY
Seymour L. Halleck, M.D.

NEUROPSYCHIATRIC FEATURES OF MEDICAL DISORDERS
James W. Jefferson, M.D., and John R. Marshall, M.D.

ADULT DEVELOPMENT: A New Dimension in Psychodynamic Theory
and Practice
Calvin A. Colarusso, M.D., and Robert A. Nemiroff, M.D.

SCHIZOPHRENIA
John S. Strauss, M.D., and William T. Carpenter, Jr., M.D.

Adult Development

A NEW DIMENSION IN PSYCHODYNAMIC THEORY AND PRACTICE

Calvin A. Colarusso, M.D.

and

Robert A. Nemiroff, M.D.

University of California—San Diego
School of Medicine
La Jolla, California

PLENUM PRESS • NEW YORK AND LONDON

Library of Congress Cataloging in Publication Data

Colarusso, Calvin A
  Adult development.

  (Critical issues in psychiatry)
  Includes index.
  1. Adulthood—Psychological aspects. 2. Psychiatry. I. Nemiroff, Robert A., joint
author. II. Title. III. Series.
BF724.5.C59   155.6   80-20250
ISBN 0-306-40619-5

©1981 Plenum Press, New York
A Division of Plenum Publishing Corporation
233 Spring Street, New York, N.Y. 10013

Printed in the United States of America

We dedicate this book to our families—our wives, Jean A. Colarusso and Barbara D. Nemiroff, and our children, Mike, Mary Ann, and Tom Colarusso, and Nancy, Susan, and Julie Nemiroff—the centers of our lives and major stimuli to our adult development.

Foreword

This volume is about the normal development of adulthood, as well as its vicissitudes and the contributions of such development to psycho-pathology. The authors are psychoanalysts of great clinical skill and perceptiveness, but while their focus is consistently a psychodynamic one, their conceptualizations about adult developmental processes are applicable to virtually all kinds of therapy.

It is extraordinary how little attention has been paid to the effects of adult developmental experience on mental development. Obviously mental structures are not static after the profound experiences of child-hood and adolescence, nor are they merely a template upon which adult experiences are processed. The authors clearly demonstrate that current adult experience always adds to, and interacts with, existing mental structure, which is itself the result of all preceding develop-ment.

After a first section in which they examine life cycle ideas on de-velopment from antiquity to the present, they present their own work as it relates to adult experience and adult development. Their hypoth-eses about the psychodynamic theory of adult development are partic-ularly creative and an enormous contribution to the psychiatric litera-ture and the clinical understanding of patients. Consistent with their views that development in adulthood is an ongoing and dynamic process, they elaborate their ideas that childhood development is fo-cused primarily on the formation of psychic structure while adult de-velopment is concerned with the continued evolution of existing struc-ture and its use. They demonstrate clearly that the developmental processes of adulthood are influenced by both the adult past *and* the childhood past, and in both instances, the process is deeply influenced by the body and physical change. A particularly important phase-specific theme of adult development is the normative crisis precipitated by the recognition and acceptance of the finiteness of time and the inevitability of personal death. These themes are elaborated and clinically applied in chapters on narcissism in the adult development of self, a chapter on myths about the adult body, male midlife crisis, parenthood, and alternative life styles.

In the third part of their book, Drs. Colarusso and Nemiroff present a method of adult developmental diagnosis and then go on to elaborate the effects of adult developmental concepts on a variety of psychotherapeutic interventions. Their theoretical concepts are then translated into practical clinical strategies to understand and treat patients with a wide variety of psychopathology. Their clinical constructs are not merely applicable to psychoanalysis or psychoanalytic psychotherapy, but also to short-term psychotherapy and other psychotherapeutic interventions. Independent of theoretical persuasion or professional title, this book will be rewarding for any mental health professional or interested lay reader, involved in the understanding of adult development themes, conflicts, or problems.

SHERWYN M. WOODS, M.D.

Acknowledgments

It is a pleasure to acknowledge the participation of the many individuals who helped us in the preparation of this book.

Sherwyn Woods, our editor, colleague, and friend, suggested the project to us. We appreciate his consistent encouragement and the high standard of scholarship that he set.

One of the most rewarding aspects of the undertaking was our collaboration with three younger colleagues: Robert Neborsky, David Talley, and Susan Zuckerman. We came to know and admire Dr. Neborsky through his work on the faculty of the Department of Psychiatry, University of California at San Diego (UCSD), where his enthusiasm and our mutual interests led eventually to collaboration. Drs. Talley and Zuckerman were junior medical students when they decided to concentrate their thesis research on adult development; their ideas and formulations contributed substantially to the chapters on the aging body and female midlife issues, respectively. We tender them warm thanks and good wishes for their futures.

During midlife, as we have stressed, time becomes an increasingly fleeting and valuable commodity. We give special thanks to Lewis Judd, Professor and Chairman of Psychiatry at UCSD, for encouraging this use of our time and for his unfailing support of our endeavor.

Behind many books, and certainly this one, is a kind of psychic organizer who helps ensure focus and consistency in the writing and preparation. Barbara Wilkes Blomgren, our good friend and neighbor, is a senior editor in the Department of Psychiatry at UCSD; we consider ourselves fortunate indeed to have had her help and advice on this project from beginning to end.

Actual writing is only one part of preparing a book for publication, and tremendous effort is required to type and retype, Xerox, write letters, check bibliographies and copyrights, and so on. For their help in these areas we thank first and foremost Rita Ballard, who is an administrative coordinator without parallel. She both encouraged us and steadfastly followed through on myriad tasks. Toward the end of our work, Debi Taylor helped enormously with copyright permissions and corrections, applying finishing touches and insuring the completion of the task. Doris Osborn and Nancy Nemiroff provided excellent typing assistance. Without their efforts we would still be in the midst of our work rather than finished.

We have had the good fortune to be associated with close friends who also share office space with us. Over weekly lunches and at other times, they gave us their ideas, encouragement, and criticisms. To Judy Braun, M.D., Brand Brickman, M.D., Esther Burstein, Ph.D., Haig Koshkarian, M.D., and Harry Woods, M.D., we express our warmest thanks.

Finally, we thank those who have taught us and those who have been taught by us, our companions in this developmental journey—particularly the clinical associates of the San Diego Psychoanalytic Institute, the residents in psychiatry at UCSD, and our patients—for providing ideas and stimulating our growth as individuals and professionals.

The permission of the following publishers to reproduce materials in this volume is gratefully acknowledged by the authors:

From E. J. Anthony and T. Benedek, *Parenthood*, p. 167. Copyright © 1970 by Little, Brown & Company. Reprinted by permission.

From Alan P. Bell and Martin S. Weinberg, *Homosexualities*, pp. 23–25, 81, 102. Copyright © 1978 by Alan P. Bell and Martin S. Weinberg. Reprinted by permission of Simon & Schuster, a Division of Gulf & Western Corporation.

From R. N. Bellah, The active life and the contemplative life. In E. H. Erikson (Ed.), *Adulthood*, p. 66. Copyright © 1978 by W. W. Norton & Company, Inc. Reprinted by permission.

From T. Benedek, Parenthood as a developmental phase. *Psychoanalytic Quarterly*, 1950, 19(1), p. 20. Copyright 1950 by the *Psychoanalytic Quarterly*. Reprinted by permission.

From E. M. Berman and H. I. Lief, Marital therapy from a psychiatric perspective: An overview (Table: "Individual and marital stages of development," p. 6). *American Journal of Psychiatry*, 1975, 132, p. 6.

Copyright © 1975 by the American Psychiatric Association. Reprinted by permission.

From J. F. Brown, *The psychodynamics of abnormal behavior*, pp. 204–206. Copyright © 1940 by McGraw-Hill Book Company. Reprinted by permission of McGraw-Hill Book Company.

From Dianne DiPrima, "Letter to John Weiners (on his 37th birthday)." In *Selected Poems, 1956–1975*, p. 251. Copyright © 1975 by North Atlantic Books, 635 Amador Street, Richmond, California 94805. Reprinted by permission of the publisher.

From Dianne DiPrima, "Poem in praise of my husband (Taos)." In *Selected Poems, 1956–1975*, p. 170. Copyright © 1975 by North Atlantic Books, 635 Amador Street, Richmond, California 94805. Reprinted by permission of the publisher.

From Dianne DiPrima, "Quartz light." In *Selected Poems, 1956–1975*, p. 190. Copyright © 1975 by North Atlantic Books, 635 Amador Street, Richmond, California 94805. Reprinted by permission of the publisher.

From E. K. Eissler, On possible effects of aging on the practice of psychoanalysis: An essay. *Journal of the Philadelphia Association for Psychoanalysis*, 1975, *11*, p. 139. Copyright 1975 by the *Journal of the Philadelphia Association for Psychoanalysis*. Reprinted by permission.

From E. H. Erikson, *Dimensions of a new identity: Jefferson lectures*, p. 124. Copyright © 1973 by W. W. Norton & Company, Inc. Reprinted by permission.

From Erik H. Erikson, *Childhood and society*, 2nd Edition, p. 274 (Figure 1), p. 268, pp. 137–138. Reprinted with the permission of W. W. Norton & Company, Inc. Copyright 1950, © 1963 by W. W. Norton & Company, Inc.

From Kathleen Fraser, "Poem in which my legs are accepted." In L. Chester & S. Barba (Eds.), *Rising tides: 20th century American women poets*, New York: Washington Square Press, 1973. Copyright 1973 by Kathleen Fraser. Reprinted by permission of author and publisher.

From Anna Freud, The concept of developmental lines. *Psychoanalytic Study of the Child*, 1963, *18*, pp. 262–264. Copyright © 1963 by International Universities Press. Reprinted by permission.

From S. Freud, Analysis terminable and interminable. In *Complete Works*, Vol. 23, Standard Edition, p. 249. Copyright 1937 by the Hogarth Press. Reprinted by permission.

lay and Norma Millay Ellis. Reprinted by permission of Norma Millay Ellis and Harper & Row, Publishers, Inc.

From B. L. Neugarten, Adult personality: Toward a psychology of the life cycle. In W. C. Sze (Ed.), *The human life cycle*, p. 384. Copyright © 1975 by Jason Aronson, Inc. Reprinted by permission.

From Gerald Pearson, *Adolescence and the conflict of generations*, pp. 21, 177. Copyright © 1958 by W. W. Norton & Company, Inc. Reprinted by permission.

From George H. Pollock, Aging or aged: Development or pathology? In Stanley I. Greenspan & George H. Pollock (Eds.), *The course of life: Psychoanalytic contributions toward understanding personality development*, Vol. III: *Adulthood and the aging process*, p. 54. Copyright 1980 by U. S. Government Printing Office, Washington, D.C. Reprinted by permission.

From D. Rapaport, On the psychoanalytic theory of motivating. In Marshall R. Jones (Ed.), *1960 Nebraska symposium on motivation*, p. 194. Copyright © 1960 by University of Nebraska Press. Reprinted by permission of University of Nebraska Press.

From Adrienne Rich, "At majority," "First things," "Thoughts on the education of daughters" (the lines "To have in this uncertain world . . . of the utmost consequence" from Wollstonecraft, *Thoughts on the education of daughters*, London, 1787), reprinted from *Snapshots of a daughter-in-law, poems 1954–1962* by Adrienne Rich, pp. 11, 47, 21–25, with the permission of W. W. Norton & Company, Inc. Copyright © 1956, 1957, 1958, 1959, 1960, 1961, 1962, 1963, 1967 by Adrienne Rich Conrad.

From T. P. Rohlen, The promise of adulthood in Japanese spiritualism. In E. H. Erikson (Ed.), *Adulthood*, p. 130. Copyright © 1978 by W. W. Norton & Company, Inc. Reprinted by permission.

From L. B. Rubin, *Women of a certain age: The midlife search for self*, p. 39–40. Copyright © 1979 by Harper & Row, Publishers, Inc. Reprinted by permission.

From Muriel Rukeyser, "Song: Remembering movies," in *The gates* (McGraw-Hill, Inc., Publishers), p. 53. Copyright © 1976 by Muriel Rukeyser. Reprinted by permission of Monica McCall, International Creative Management, as agent for the author.

From Susan Fromberg Schaeffer, "Age" (Excerpted from "The Housewife") in *Granite lady* (Macmillan, Inc., Publishers), p. 102. Copyright © 1974 by Susan Fromberg Schaeffer. Reprinted by permission of Russell & Bolkening, Inc., as agents for the author.

From Anne Sexton, "Little girl, my stringbean, my lovely women," in *Live or die* by Anne Sexton, pp. 62–65. Copyright © 1966 by Anne Sexton. Reprinted by permission of Houghton Mifflin Company, Publishers.

From Anne Sexton, "Two sons," in *Live or die* by Anne Sexton, p. 33. Copyright © 1966 by Anne Sexton. Reprinted by permission of Houghton Mifflin Company, Publishers.

From M. Shane, Countertransference and the developmental approach. *Psychoanalysis and Contemporary Thought*, 1980, *3*, pp. 196, 208. Reprinted by permission of author.

From M. Shane, A rationale for teaching analytic technique based on a developmental orientation and approach. *International Journal of Psycho-Analysis*, 1977, *58*(95), pp. 97, 98, 100, 102, 103–104. Copyright © 1977 by the *International Journal of Psycho-Analysis*. Reprinted by permission.

From Judith Stevens-Long, *Adult life*, pp. 5–6, 115, 142–143. Reprinted by permission of Mayfield Publishing Company. Copyright © 1979 by Mayfield Publishing Company.

From George E. Vaillant, *Adaptation to life*, Table 3, p. 80; Table 4, p. 275; Figure 3, p. 331; excerpt, p. 41. Copyright © 1977 by George E. Vaillant. Reprinted by permission of Little, Brown and Company, Publishers.

From Laurens vander Post, *A portrait of Japan*, p. 129. Copyright 1968 by The Hogarth Press, LTD. Reprinted by permission.

From A. Van Gennep, *The rites of passage*, pp. 2–3, 43–44, 107. Reprinted by permission of the University of Chicago Press. Copyright © 1960 by the University of Chicago Press.

CALVIN COLARUSSO
ROBERT NEMIROFF

Department of Psychiatry
School of Medicine
University of California, San Diego

Contents

Introduction
Adult Development
AN OVERVIEW

The study of the life span is reminiscent of a fifteenth-century map of the world. Europe, the origin of the map, is carefully detailed. All the shapes and proportions are recognizable in the context of current knowledge. Like the study of childhood, the territory looks familiar. On the other side of the world, China—like the psychology of later life—is partially mapped. In the middle, however, stretch vast, unexplored territories. Odd shapes and sizes, fanciful names, and vague outlines are everywhere.

Those who study adulthood quickly discover the limits of our information as did those early cartographers. Little is known about adulthood, and especially about the middle years, from the twenties to age sixty-five. But the unknown lures us and we have a sense of adventure. It is exciting to be among the first to explore the area. We know enough to realize that there is much more to learn—enough to motivate the most energetic and imaginative among us.

Judith Stevens-Long, 1979, pp. 5–6

Like Stevens-Long, we feel a kinship with the early cartographers and see our efforts as tentative steps into the essentially uncharted territory of adulthood. Our focus of study is primarily the individual. Like Freud, Erikson, Piaget, and other developmentalists, we inquire into the lives of single human beings and then build a general theory from our observations, using our psychoanalytic orientation and clinical experience as the main investigative tools. Although this approach places us in eminent company, it separates us from those investigators who study groups of people and insist on statistical validation of their findings. However, the two approaches need not be seen as contradictory or mutually exclusive; they can serve well to complement one another.

The unmapped territory is large enough for cartographers with instruments of all kinds.

Our main interest is the elaboration of the normal development of adulthood. A basic premise of our work is that developmental processes occur throughout the life span. The adult, therefore, is understood to be a dynamic, constantly changing organism. In our efforts to contribute to a psychodynamic theory of adulthood, we have tried to formulate a set of working hypotheses about the nature of development in the normal adult and to describe the intrapsychic events that partly determine and are the result of that development. Because our focus is the normal adult, our work may be of interest to professionals and intelligent laymen alike. Certainly, we intend to address ourselves to all readers who are curious about themselves and those around them.

First and foremost, we are clinicians, spending most of our time treating children and adults. Our data come primarily, but not exclusively, from our patients. Clinical work gives us the privilege of studying the human mind in detail through the fine and powerful microscope provided by the analytical method, and this book includes many clinical examples illustrating the major concepts. Because we are also introspective and curious about the developmental processes in ourselves and in those around us, additional and important sources of information have been observations of ourselves, families, friends, and acquaintances.

In addition to elaborating a theory of normal adult development, we apply the ideas to clinical work with patients, believing that a knowledge and understanding of the developmental processes in the adult has great relevance for the clinician regardless of his professional discipline, level of training, or theoretical orientation. This book is not intended only for analysts, nor is it primarily about analysis; adult-developmental ideas can affect all forms of therapeutic effort, from crisis intervention, through brief- and long-term psychotherapy, to psychoanalysis. Students of social work, psychology, psychiatry, and related disciplines should find these concepts applicable to their work with patients. This effort may also have relevance for intelligent laypersons who are inquisitive about themselves and those around them. In essence, we are attempting to describe, from our vantage point, a view of human nature, eliciting the themes common to us all.

The third focus of attention is the educational process in adulthood. Although we write specifically about the education of mental-health professionals, our postulate is that learning in adulthood, as in childhood, is a developmental experience and should be understood as such by student and teacher alike, regardless of the field of study.

THE QUESTION OF REDUCTIONISM

When adult behavior is explained on the basis of infantile experience—an aspect of psychoanalytic theory—critics claim that such explanations are reductionistic. On the other hand, when adult behavior is explained on the basis of current experience, without accounting for genetic factors, charges of superficiality are advanced. We do not question the great importance of childhood experience in forming the adult personality. Indeed, it is a tenet of our work that childhood developmental themes continue to play central roles in the adult. In particular, we agree with the psychoanalytic observation that behind every adult neurosis is an unresolved infantile neurosis. But we do believe that too little attention has been paid to the effects of *adult* experience on mental development. A natural corollary of the belief that developmental processes continue throughout life is the idea that adult experience is a major determinant of further development.

If behavior and mental development are explained in terms of infantile *or* adult experience, a simplistic theory must result; a more comprehensive understanding is likely to emerge from attempts to integrate the effects of both. Because this book is about adult development it may seem that adult factors are overemphasized. That is not our intent; we hypothesize that current experience *always* adds to and interacts with existing mental structure, which is itself the result of all preceding development.

THE ORGANIZATION OF THE BOOK

Of the three parts into which the book is divided, the first is a summation of ideas on development from antiquity to the present. In Part II we present our own work as it related to various aspects of adult experience, and in Part III we describe the relevance of those ideas to clinical work and the education of mental-health professionals.

Part I

Chapter 1: The Life Cycle in Antiquity: Some Images of Adulthood in Various Cultures and Religions

Ancient civilizations, both Western and Eastern, had sophisticated ideas about adult development which continue to have relevance for current thinking, and we present briefly ideas ranging across the Judeo-Christian, Greco-Roman, and Oriental traditions.

Chapter 2: The Pioneer Developmentalists

The foundation for much current adult-developmental theory is based on the work of four men. In Chapter 2 we present the major developmental ideas of Van Gennep, Freud, Jung, and Erikson. Van Gennep, an anthropologist, was interested in those ceremonies that define developmental milestones in the lives of individuals and societies. He called them *rites of passage*. A contemporary of Freud, he underscored the universality of developmental themes and experiences. Freud, whose focus was the individual, began the definition of the developmental stages of childhood. The libidinal stages he described—oral, anal, oedipal, latency, adolescence—provided a framework for the exploration of the developmental evolution of the human organism and stimulated those who followed, including Jung and Erikson.

It is not generally recognized that Carl Jung was a pioneer in adult development. Whereas Freud focused on the developmental sequences in childhood, Jung was interested in the developmental phenomena of middle and later life as well.

Eric Erikson, the most contemporary of the pioneers, was the first to define a developmental outline for the entire life cycle. His eight stages of life are a significant theoretical advance because for the first time developmental concepts are validated for the entire life span. Our own work and that of other adult developmentalists rests squarely on Erikson's concepts and builds from them.

Chapter 3: Contemporary Adult Developmentalists

The modern developmentalists whose work is presented in this chapter, by focusing their efforts on the adult, have begun for the first time the delineation of a comprehensive theory of adulthood. Pioneers in their own right, Roger Gould, Daniel Levinson, Robert Lifton, Bernice Neugarten, George Pollock, and George Vaillant have made major contributions to our understanding. Their backgrounds and approaches vary, but they share the beliefs that development is lifelong and adulthood is a time of dynamic growth and change. They are the current cartographers, filling in the blank spots on the map.

Part II

Chapter 4: Hypotheses about the Psychodynamic Theory of Adult Development

We have formulated seven hypotheses about development in adulthood: (1) The nature of the developmental process is basically the same in the adult as in the child. (2) Development in adulthood is an ongoing, dynamic process. (3) Whereas child development is focused primarily in the formation of psychic structure, adult development is concerned with the continued evolution of existing structure and with its use. (4) The fundamental developmental issues of childhood continue as central aspects of adult life but in altered form. (5) The developmental processes in adulthood are influenced by the adult past as well as the childhood past. (6) Development in adulthood, as in childhood, is deeply influenced by the body and physical change. (7) A central, phase-specific theme of adult development is the normative crisis precipitated by the recognition and acceptance of the finiteness of time and the inevitability of personal death. For the reader with a limited amount of time, perhaps Chapter 4 is the best place to begin.

Chapter 5: Narcissism in the Adult Development of the Self

The concept of the self has recently come into prominence as a theoretical tool for explaining behavior. In this chapter we try to describe the major adult experiences that determine the continued evolvement of the self, focusing particularly on the role of narcissism in that process. The concept of authenticity is used to characterize the mature adult self because it describes the capacity to accept what is genuine within the self and the outer world regardless of the narcissistic injury involved. Confrontation with the developmental tasks of midlife precipitates a normal narcissistic regression leading to a reemergence of aspects of infantile grandiosity. The reworking and eventual integration of these powerful feelings are integral parts of normal development at midlife.

Chapter 6: Myths about the Aging Body

Although research has not yet yielded a satisfactory fund of information about the normal biological and maturational events of adulthood, a survey of the literature indicates that emerging data are calling into question many heretofore accepted ideas. To the extent that further research will substantiate such findings, many current "facts" are likely in the future to be recognized as myths; for example; that the menopausal syndrome is caused by estrogen deficiency; postmenopausal women cannot enjoy sex because of the physiological and psychological effects of estrogen withdrawal; a decrease in testosterone levels is responsible for the decline in sexual functioning in older men; impotence is a natural consequence of aging; intelligence reaches a peak in the twenties and then declines at a steady rate; the aging brain loses weight and neurons and demonstrates inevitable senile changes; or that the adult brain is a finished product, incapable of structural change.

Although some degree of sexual and intellectual decline is an inevitable consequence of aging, most of these changes are caused by poor health and social or cultural factors rather than the physiological changes of aging per se. The widely held view that the elderly are essentially asexual and doomed to senility is biologically unsound, but can become a more-or-less self-fulfilling prophecy.

Chapter 7: Male Midlife Crisis: The Gauguin Syndrome, Myth and Reality

The great Postimpressionist painter Paul Gauguin has come to personify the male in midlife crisis. Supposedly, he suddenly left his wife and children and ran off to paint naked women in paradise. The reality was quite different, and much more mundane. Using Gauguin as an example of the distortions and confusion that characterize much current thinking about midlife crisis, we describe the range of change that takes place in middle age, most of which is transitional rather than critical. In contrast, then, we present a detailed clinical case example of a genuine midlife crisis.

Chapter 8: The Father at Midlife: Crisis and Growth of Paternal Identity

Midlife is a particularly formative time in the evolution of paternal identity because of the unique phase-specific interaction between issues of midlife development in the father and adolescent development in his children. Paternal reaction to adolescent children is more than a simple response to the adolescent process; it is also an expression of powerful developmental forces within the parent which are impinged upon by the adolescent offspring.

The experience of fatherhood is described as a dynamic one, undergoing continuous intrapsychic evolution through young adulthood, midlife, and the later years. In fact, the experience of being a father at 25 is so different than at 45 or 55 that the only similarity from an intrapsychic standpoint is the designation *father*. Being a father can result in the emergence of new capacities. For example. we relate paternal generativity (Erikson's concept of caring for the next generation) to relinquishing control over the lives of adolescent offspring and the sublimation of feelings of weakness, passivity, helplessness, and rage that are engendered in the process.

Chapter 9: Female Midlife Issues in Prose and Poetry

If the study of midlife is a frontier, the study of women in midlife is the remotest outpost on that frontier. In this chapter we try to frame research questions, capture the essence of feminine experience as expressed by women writers and poets, and present the sparse research results that are available. The material is organized around the fundamental themes of midlife: the body, object relations, work, time, and death. Each of those areas presents special problems for women. Because prevailing sociocultural views equate femininity and sexual desirability with a youthful body, many middle-aged women experience more painful, more prolonged preoccupation with the physical signs of aging than do their male counterparts.

In midlife parents age, children grow and leave, and sexual, marital, and career needs change. Women may have more difficulty than men have in achieving autonomy from parents because their attachment is grounded in the longer and more intense identification mothers have with daughters than with sons. Those feelings often peak, because of the aging or death of parents, at the same time that intense ties to one's own children are threatened by adolescent separation. Contrary to popular belief, many women do not experience only a sense of loss when their children leave; in addition many feel decided relief and excitement over the opportunity to begin a new phase of life. The anticipation of a new career at midlife may bring genuine pleasure and fulfillment, but, because of conflicted personal and societal attitudes and unrealistic expectations, considerable pain and disappointment as well.

Women experience the passage of time with keen intensity, differently from the way men experience it. The end of the reproductive life of the women occurs in midlife, bringing with it a jarring reappraisal of time spent and time left. In most other ways, however, particularly in regard to career, socially defined standards of temporal appropriateness are based on the male life cycle, not the realities of feminine midlife existence. These and other factors characterize what is a uniquely feminine attitude toward time and aging.

Chapter 10: Difficult Questions and Variations in Lifestyles

In this chapter we address questions of the nature, universality, and variation in development. Certain aspects of development, particularly those precipitated by genetically determined maturational events, are inescapable and universal, but there is infinite variation within the basic experiences common to all.

Development is a cross-cultural phenomenon in which each culture unconsciously structures its child-rearing practices to produce adults who can function productively and pass traditions on to the next generation. Universal developmental themes also cut across class lines and levels of society.

Normality is difficult to define and constantly changing in any given culture, but normal development, as we understand that phrase, is most likely to occur when individuals in passing from stage to stage engage in the successive developmental tasks to the fullest.

Western culture is currently in a state of flux that is likely to engender widespread repercussions in developmental processes. In attempting to relate adult-developmental concepts to the revolutionary changes in attitudes and behavior that exist today, we discuss such contemporary issues as divorce and remarriage, the single state, and the effects of homosexual thoughts, feelings, and actions on development. Our basic attitude is one of open inquiry. We do not know the long-range effects of any of these increasingly common lifestyles on development in adulthood, but we do know that the effects will be complex and profound and confront the psychodynamically oriented researcher with many difficult questions for which there are no ready answers.

Part III

Chapter 11: The Adult-Developmental Diagnosis

Developmental concepts alter the diagnostic process with adult patients because they influence the therapist's attitude about the patient and his problems, the collection and recording of data, and the diagnostic and treatment formulations. The purpose of doing such an evaluation is to obtain a clear understanding of the normal and deviant developmental factors from childhood and adulthood that underlie the patient's healthy growth and symptoms. This developmental construction, coupled with a psychodynamic understanding of the patient's intrapsychic conflicts, physical state, and environmental interactions, provides the information necessary to make a comprehensive diagnostic and treatment formulation.

In this chapter we present a comprehensive outline of an adult-developmental evaluation, a theoretical rationale for the gathering and organization of the material, and a detailed case illustration. We also include an outline of a developmental history for the entire life cycle and consider developmental themes along developmental lines, using a concept originated by Anna Freud (1965) in regard to children.

Chapter 12: The Effects of Adult-Developmental Concepts on Psychotherapy

The developmental orientation has important implications for psychotherapy because it provides the therapist with a new framework from which to view the adult. A patient of any age is understood to be in the midst of dynamic change. Thus older patients, formerly thought to be unsuitable for exploratory psychotherapy, are now viewed as potential candidates. Furthermore, the developmental orientation emphasizes the potential for healthy development. Pathology, then, is redefined primarily as deviation from normal development, an outgrowth of inadequate developmental functioning. The goal of treatment thus becomes not symptom removal but the elimination of blocks to the still-evolving personality and to the course of current and future development.

The conduct of psychotherapy is discussed in relation to the major adult-developmental themes outlined in Chapter 4, and clinical examples are used to illustrate how developmental issues relating to childhood, the adult body, thoughts of time and death, and the adult past are expressed in therapy.

The therapist's attitude toward his patient is described through the term *developmental resonance*—the therapeutic capacity to share, respect, understand, and value the thoughts and feelings of patients of all ages because of the implicit awareness on the part of the therapist that he either has experienced or likely will experience something akin to what the patient is experiencing.

Chapter 13: Psychotherapeutic Technique and Development

Morton Shane, a psychoanalyst working in Los Angeles, has been a pioneer in applying adult-developmental concepts to therapeutic technique. Using his work and our own, we describe developmental aspects of free association, nonverbal communication, outside motivation and information, transference, resistance and defense, reconstructions, countertransference, and termination.

In essence, the ability to free-associate is a developmental process that grows and changes during the course of treatment. Patients must learn the technique, and their abilities to utilize it differ. A developmental orientation suggests that the modes of communication between adult patient and therapist may be broadened; for example, a rationale is given, along with examples, for looking at pictures drawn by an adult patient, or examining a work of art. Also, gestures and other forms of nonverbal communication are not discouraged but are used as vehicles for understanding. Although it is generally recognized that children are incapable of communicating symbolically in words alone, it is not as understood that many adults are also limited in their ability to communicate verbally and must use other forms of expression.

The term *working alliance* refers to the rational rapport that develops between therapist and patient. As with free association, that rapport is understood as a developmental process occurring within the therapeutic relationship. The ability to form and sustain a working relationship will vary from patient to patient and depend in part upon progression along the developmental line of caring for the self. The working alliance is also subject to regression and fixation; in all forms of dynamic psychotherapy it should be observed, explained, and analyzed as it develops.

Because adult patients are involved in vital, intimate relationships with other adults, the developmentally oriented therapist is not distressed by the recognition that motivation and the working alliance are strongly influenced by others. The intimacy and trust implicit in the working alliance itself may be viewed as a threat by others, such as the patient's spouse, for those attitudes are also an integral part of marriage. The recognition of the similarities allows the therapist to empathize with the spouse and explore with the patient (and the spouse if necessary) how the treatment relationship can be used by the patient to enhance (or inhibit) intimacy in other relationships.

The concept of transference, too, is broadened by developmental principles. Transference is understood to be a special kind of attitude toward a person in the present which is based on experiences with others in the past. From a developmental standpoint, this new attitude does not emanate solely from the childhood past but from *all* past phases of development. The situation may be further complicated by the fact that the parents of childhood and other significant figures may be alive and influential in the present. Moreover, the adult patient may use the therapist as a transference object in ways not possible for younger patients; a prime example would be a son or daughter transference.

By using a developmental perspective with regard to defenses, the therapist can better organize his understanding of a patient's resistances and select an appropriate response. It is generally agreed that resistances and defenses are selectively interpreted in exploratory therapy. The clear identification of phase-specific and phase-approved defenses helps the therapist plan his interventions, because they are less frequently in need of interpretation than more primitive or maladaptive defenses.

Reconstructions, the deductions of patient and therapist about important events and feelings that must have occurred in the patient's past, are an important part of exploratory psychotherapy. Thinking developmentally is a great help to the clinician in reconstructing the patient's unique life experience.

In relation to countertransference, the developmental approach emphasizes the complex, multiple layers of representations from the therapist's past and present. If the therapist is understood to be a still-developing individual, in the midst of his own current developmental conflict, each therapeutic encounter becomes a vehicle for growth or regression.

Among the criteria most commonly used to determine readiness for termination are symptom relief, structural change, transference resolution, and improvement in self-esteem. The developmental approach adds one important dimension, namely, the resumption of normal development. As a criterion for termination, the resumption of normal development is a broader notion underlying all the others.

Chapter 14: Clinical Applications: An Adult-Developmental Approach to Hysterical Psychopathology

The core hypothesis of this chapter is that midlife developmental pressures can strongly influence the onset, course, and treatment of psychopathology. Here clinical examples are used to demonstrate the relevance of adult-developmental concepts to the diagnosis, understanding, and short-term treatment of hysterical syndromes. Because of a combination of denial, repression, and somatization, the clinician often has little therapeutic leverage with such patients in a short-term situation. But many patients readily comprehend and are willing to work with the therapist in assessing the basic issues of midlife. Moreover, successful short-term psychotherapy does not depend upon in-depth reconstructions or interpretations but in the ability to free the patient enough to proceed with adult development without regression or fixation, a goal achieved with each of the four patients presented in the chapter.

Chapter 15: Adult Development and the Educational Process

The implications of the developmental orientation for the educational process are myriad, affecting what is taught and how it is communicated as well as the roles of student and teacher. Although we speak specifically about the education of mental-health professionals, many of the ideas are applicable to any learning situation.

In planning a developmental curriculum, primary emphasis should be placed on teaching the theory of normal development through the life cycle. Those concepts may then be related to psychopathology, diagnosis, and treatment. The study of the life cycle should include lectures, seminars, and direct observations, both serial and longitudinal, of children, adults, and families.

When the major psychopathological processes of childhood and adulthood are presented, the student is helped to grasp the correlation between adult and child psychopathology and to begin defining the similarities and differences between normal and pathological processes throughout the life cycle.

A spiral curriculum, as described in the report of the Conference on Psychoanalytic Education and Research (1974), can be used. Basic concepts are introduced and then elaborated upon throughout the training years, allowing for continual integration of new ideas with older ones. Whenever possible, courses should be taught jointly by male and female instructors who have treated adults and children.

Chapter 15 includes a description of a developmental sequence for the student, incorporating the educational experience as an integral part of young-adult development. Adult students must balance educational demands with those relating to intimacy, marriage, family, and so on. We give as examples the experiences of four female psychiatry residents, all involved in balancing their desire for professional training with their desire for motherhood.

In a section subtitled "Psychotherapy—The Developmental Crucible for Student and Supervisor," we discuss the effects of the supervisory triangle (student, supervisor, patient) on both student and supervisor. Because the student-therapist must use himself as the instrument of observation and treatment, his current intrapsychic equilibrium is upset. Feelings of inexperience and inadequacy may cause the apprentice to idealize his supervisor in the initial phase of their mentee–mentor relationship. Conversely, becoming a supervisor is

every bit as much of a developmental experience as becoming a therapist, and we describe the developmental line of becoming a supervisor,
beginning with one's first experience being supervised. We note the
powerful narcissistic gratifications involved and the pitfalls that can appear if both student and teacher do not recognize the complexity of
their relationship.

In closing the chapter, and the book, we describe our experience
as teachers of development to first-year psychiatric residents and psychoanalytic candidates. We teach a course on the normal development
of adulthood to third- and fourth-year psychoanalytic candidates at the
San Diego Psychoanalytic Institute, and we include here a detailed bib-
liography and course outline, along with two sample clinical presentations illustrating the use of adult-developmental concepts by the clinical associates of the institute. We also introduce the developmental
framework to first-year psychiatric residents in the Department of Psychiatry at the University of California at San Diego. The goals of the series of developmental case conferences are to introduce concepts of
normal child and adult development, to illustrate those concepts with
case material, and to relate them to diagnostic and therapeutic work
with patients.

REFERENCES

Conference on Psychoanalytic Education and Research. Commission IX, "Child Anal-
    ysis." New York: American Psychoanalytic Association, 1974.
Freud, A. *Normality and pathology in childhood: Assessments of development.* New York: Inter-
    national Universities Press, 1965.
Stevens-Long, J. *Adult life: Developmental process.* Palo Alto, Calif.: Mayfield, 1979.

I

ORIGINS

1

The Life Cycle in Antiquity

SOME IMAGES OF ADULTHOOD IN VARIOUS CULTURES AND RELIGIONS

And one man in his time plays many parts,
His acts being seven ages. At first the infant,
Mewling and puking in the nurse's arms.
Then the whining schoolboy, with his satchel
And shining morning face, creeping like snail
Unwillingly to school. And then the lover,
Sighing like furnace, with a woeful ballad
Made to his mistress' eyebrow. Then a soldier,
Full of strange oaths and bearded like the pard,
Jealous in honor, sudden and quick in quarrel,
Seeking the bubble reputation
Even in the cannon's mouth. And then the justice,
In fair round belly with good capon lined,
With eyes severe and beard of formal cut,
Full of wise saws and modern instances,
And so he plays his part. The sixth age shifts
Into the lean and slippered Pantaloon
With spectacles on nose and pouch on side,
His youthful hose, well saved, a world too wide
For his shrunk shank, and his big manly voice,
Turning again toward childish treble, pipes
And whistles in his sound. Last scene of all
That ends this strange eventful history,
Is second childishness and mere oblivion,
Sans teeth, sans eyes, sans taste, sans everything.

Shakespeare, *As You Like It*, II, vii, 142–166

Human beings have always had a profound need for a comprehensive
perspective of their lives, and writings from diverse cultures and reli-

3

gions speak to these issues in terms that are astonishingly consistent with contemporary thought.

Although social scientists have only recently begun to study distinct phases of adult development, the human life cycle[1] has been a subject of interest and concern to students of human nature from the beginning of recorded history. For instance, the Greek poet and philosopher Solon (639–559 B.C.) divided the course of a man's life into seven-year periods and indicated the growth appropriate to each in a life span encompassing seven decades. He described six periods of adulthood and assigned appropriate developmental tasks to each, such as learning to use one's capacities to the fullest, becoming a husband and father, and increasing in virtue. When the course of adulthood is smooth, "tongue and mind for fourteen years together [are] at their best." That accomplished, a man departs on the ebb tide of death having remained nimble in speech and wit for his allotted time.

Solon's near-contemporary in China, Confucius (551–479 B.C.), described his personal yet representative journey succinctly, indicating that at 15 he had set his heart upon learning; at 30 planted his feet firmly upon the ground; at 40 no longer suffered from perplexities; at 50 knew the biddings of heaven; and at 60 could "follow the dictates of his own heart, for what [he] desired no longer overstepped the boundaries of right."

Gradually these developmental sequences were translated into cultural and religious expectations. For example, during the first centuries A.D. the oral laws of the Hebrews were written into the Talmud. Prescribed there are successive stages of maturation in the faith which are themselves an outline of the life cycle: learning the laws, assuming moral responsibility, pursuing scholarly understanding, marrying, pursuing an occupation, attaining full capability, reaching understanding, giving counsel, becoming an elder, and, finally, bending under the weight of the years and passing from the world.

If we now leap across the centuries to the present and examine the work of a prominent contemporary developmentalist, Daniel Levinson, we find a remarkable compatibility with the observations of the early Greeks, Chinese, and Hebrews. His version of the male life cycle (he did not study women) ascribes the first 15 to 20 years of life to childhood. During early adulthood, which lasts about 15 years, a young

---

[1] By the term *life cycle* we mean the course an individual follows beginning with birth, including the experiences of all the intervening years, and ending with death.

man enters the adult world, mates, and pursues an occupation. Although by 30 a man has attained his strength and found his place, he has not yet achieved his most mature capabilities. With Solon, Confucius, and the Talmud, Levinson describes the middle-adulthood years, from about 40 to 60, as the period of greatest actualization of one's capacities and contributions to society, notwithstanding some attenuation of physical energy. Late adulthood begins around the seventh decade of life. Whereas Solon described this final stage as a time of inevitable decline, Levinson, Confucius, and talmudic scholars construed that era as having cumulative significance for the individual's life, as an opportunity to transcend through wisdom born of experience the old conflicts between desire and morality, between self and other, and between individual and society.

THE LIFE SPAN AND THE LIFE CYCLE

It is important to view the human life cycle not only from the perspective of individual potentialities but from the standpoint of the life span as well, since the gradual increase in life expectancy has had a determining effect upon the life cycle itself and on the way it has been understood and interpreted. It is generally accepted by anthropologists that the human species has existed for between half a million and three million years; yet only five or ten thousand years ago humans were leading precarious, unsettled lives in small societies and surviving by hunting, fishing, and gathering food. The development of agriculture marked the formation of more stable societies and technological progress. In primitive hunting/gathering societies only half the population reached age 20, and not more than 10% survived beyond 40. Thus middle adulthood is a relatively recent human experience, since primitive man had completed his essential reproductive, parental, and occupational functions by the time he reached 40. Moreover, it must be recognized that the experience of middle age is not a common one in many parts of the world today. In Pakistan, with both a high birthrate and extreme poverty, only 17% of the population is over 40 years old; Ethiopia and Bangladesh have even lower percentages of people living after 40 (Levinson, Darrow, Klein, Levinson, & McKee, 1978). Thus, viewed against the perspective of evolution, and considering evidence from the poorer countries of today, we can appreciate the fact that adulthood—that is, the second half of life (from 30 on)—has been part of human experience for a remarkably short time.

Although mankind has been interested in the notion of his development for several thousand years, the *scientific study* of the life cycle is a recent event as the following demonstrates. Aries (1962) has shown that the idea of *childhood* did not exist in medieval society. Both the term and the concept *adolescence* were first popularized in 1904 by Hall, who did the same for *senescence* in 1922 (Jordan, 1978). As recently as 1968 the *International Encyclopedia of the Social Sciences* had articles on adolescence and aging, but none on adulthood (Jordan, 1978). Similarly, until recently there was not even a term for adulthood in the Russian language (Malia, 1978). Thus, although poets and philosophers have long offered perspectives on the span of a human life, scientific scholars have just begun to focus on the phases of the human life cycle, particularly adulthood. We are indebted to our forebears for their insights, but are left with the fascinating task of elaborating the structure of the life cycle using the tools of modern science.

IMAGES OF ADULTHOOD

To provide a setting for the coming chapters, we want to familiarize the reader somewhat with thoughts about the life cycle from various major cultures and religions. In surveying briefly the variety of images of adulthood reflected in literary and philosophical writings from other times and cultures, we rely heavily on the anthology *Adulthood*, edited by Erikson (1978). Although the sources represented in that volume are diverse (including psychoanalytic, medical, literary, dramatic, personal, historical, and religious material), all produce evidence for the existence of broad universal outlines of the human life cycle and concepts of adulthood which are consistent across cultures and historical time.

We find the following themes consistently present in these writings and in our own experience:

1. A comprehensive, chronological life cycle can be described.
2. Adulthood is not static; the adult is in a constant state of dynamic change and flux, always in a state of "becoming" or "finding the way."
3. Development in adulthood is contiguous with that in childhood and old age.

4. There is continual need to define the adult self, especially with regard to the integrity of the inner man vs. his external environment.

5. Adults must come to terms with their limited span and individual mortality. A preoccupation with time is an expression of these concerns.

6. The development and maintenance of the adult body and its relationship to the mind is a universal preoccupation.

7. Narcissism, that is, love of self vs. responsibility to the society in which one lives and the individuals in that society toward whom one bears responsibility as an adult, is a central issue in all civilized cultures.

It is beyond our scope here to describe the cultural sources of these themes in detail, but we offer the following examples, illustrating their relation to adult development, to suggest how various peoples have dealt with the life cycle and conceptualized the process of maturing.

CONFUCIANISM

In the late Chow period, anarchy prevailed in China as ambitious feudal retainers overthrew their lords and pursued their own needs and goals. Appalled by the political and social conditions of the time, Confucius and his disciples worked to restore the moral order. To their way of thinking, adulthood was not a state of attainment but the continual process of cultivating one's humanity. In their scheme, education in the home began at the age of six; at seven the sexes were separated; etiquette was taught from age eight; arithmetic from age nine. Formal schooling began at 10, and by 13 the youth studied music, poetry, dance, ritual, archery, and horsemanship. When a man reached 20, the rite of the capping ceremony marked his coming of age. In his thirties, having married and become a father, he was a fully participating member of society. Normally the career of scholar/official began at 40, by which age a man was considered mature and responsible. By 50 he would reach the height of his public service and function at that level until past 70 (Tu, 1978).

Essential to the Confucian concept of the adult man is the metaphor of *the Way*, a term describing the process of maturation involving continuous effort toward self-realization. A sense of inner direction

must be endlessly discovered and put into action. The Way is insepara-
ble from the person; it is experienced as an internal presence. It is
never perceived as an external path; it is not based on social norms and
so cannot be used as a measure of worldly success or construed as ad-
herence to a set of directives. Tu (1978) describes the development of
the maturing adult in Confucian terms as he who

> never ceases to "set his heart on the Way." Nor does he relax his "firm
> grasp on virtue." Indeed, he always endeavors to "rely on humanity and to
> find recreation in the arts" so that he can broaden himself with "culture"
> . . . and refine himself with "ritual" . . . His "ambition" is to become a
> "man of humanity" who, "wishing to establish his own character, also es-
> tablishes the character of others, and wishing to be prominent himself, also
> helps others to be prominent." His learning is "for the sake of himself" . . .
> and he does not regard himself as an "instrument" . . . , for his mode of ex-
> istence is to be an end rather than a tool for any external purpose . . . . In
> fact, no matter how hard he works and how much distance he covers, a
> true man is, as it were, all the time on the Way. (p. 115)

The Confucian version of the Golden Rule, that one ought never
do unto others what one would not want done unto oneself, retains
the Eastern emphasis on self-cultivation as the pathway whereby a person ultimately manifests genuine humanity, or human-ness, in relation
to others. The culmination of mastering the art of living well is the ability to die with grace and acceptance.

Confucianism teaches the development of the body as well as intellectual and ethical growth. The involvement of the body is so integral to the Confucian ideal that the Way has been characterized as "the
learning of the body and mind," and mastery of the six arts that constitute the core of Confucian teaching requires harmony between the two:
archery and charioteering; ritual and music; calligraphy and arithmetic.
Literally, one who has achieved humanity *embodies* the Way.

The Confucian philosophy and its perspective on adulthood return
always to the Way as a process of becoming, one of the oldest representations of the idea that individual human beings develop in mind
and body throughout their lives.

JAPANESE SPIRITUALISM

Age and considerations of time hold central places in ancient Japanese spiritualism and in the traditional culture of Japan. Experience is

respected, the elderly are well cared for, and age is viewed as a measure of wisdom. Ruth Benedict pointed out that the life cycle in Japan
is conceived of as U-shaped. The high points of the U represent the
greater ease, gratification, and freedom of both childhood and old age:

CHILDHOOD   OLD AGE

ADULTHOOD

   In the traditional view, adulthood is arranged so as to lead to a satisfactory old age (Rohlen, 1978). Age becomes an important organizing
principle, and Japanese leaders, whether politicians, businessmen,
scholars, or artists, are generally older than their counterparts in the
Western societies. Classically, the Japanese view adulthood as a
process demanding considerable effort and attention wherein one becomes more and more free of the "self," culminating in the ease, creativity, and wisdom of old age.

   Concern with time, age, and change pervades the Japanese culture. For example, to be spoken properly, the language requires precise
knowledge of the relative ages of the parties (Rohlen, 1978). According
to vander Post (1968), the language seems to be organized on the basis
of potential states of being, possibility, and moods, and the verbs describe things that have not yet happened, might happen, are about to
happen, are happening, or have happened—" . . . a tongue full of allu-
sion, suggestion, mood, and association of endless poetic nuance and
possibility, which is the despair of the abstract thinkers and logical pos-
itivists of our world" (p. 108). Even in dress there is a precise relation
of pattern and color to fine gradations in age.

   The contrast with the Western emphasis on self-aggrandizement
and technological estrangement from nature is obvious in the following
description of the Japanese appreciation of the seasonal qualities of living and the role of time in individual development.

> The Japanese inhabit a cultural world profoundly concerned with the
> turn of seasons, of years, of whole lives. Time is a flow of change that is es-
> sentially universal in its pattern. Just as each season has its character and its
> particular beauty, so each part of life should be accepted and appreciated
> for what it brings. . . . acceptance and appreciation of this kind of nature-
> given reality, a form of truth that not only surrounds human existence but
> *is* human existence, involves a submission of the "self" . . . Giving up self-
> centered awareness is far from an easy task. Life, however, is a stern and
> implacable teacher, and part of the fascination of the Japanese view of bio-

graphical time is that it is at once fatalistic (nature has its way) and yet, contrary to our understanding of that fatalism, simultaneously preoccupied with the challenge and potential for human perfection contained in the submission of "self" to a greater reality. Acceptance of aging, for example, brings the person into closer contact with all natural change. This to the Japanese is a form of religious fulfillment. (Rohlen, 1978, p. 130)

The Western term "adulthood" finds no easy translation in the Japanese language. Whereas the American ideal of development is for a child to become increasingly independent of others, in Japan the infant is seen as separate to begin with and needing to be drawn into ever greater interdependency with others (Caudill & Weinstein, 1969). A high compliment paid to mature individuals, usually to people in their forties or older, is, "For him, the process of becoming human is complete." The major characteristics of such an individual are his empathy and openness to others (Rohlen, 1978). Leaders are evaluated in terms of the degree to which they have developed the insight, self-control, and interpersonal skills associated with such human-ness.

Vander Post (1968) cites a favorite story to illustrate the Japanese ideal of humanity and its relation to the needs of others:

> Two Zen monks were walking in the country after a flood. They came to a place where the road was cut by a torrent and the bridge washed away. On the far side a girl in distress called out to the monks, begging them to help her across. Monk A immediately, Zen-like, rolled up his sleeves, girded up his kimono, waded across, put the girl on his shoulder, carried her over the torrent and put her down. Then he and Monk B crossed over themselves and continued on their way. For the first seven miles, however, Monk B, who had done nothing, was deep in thought and silent. Suddenly he said, "Brother, I am very worried. We are holy men and today you have broken your vows by touching a woman and carrying her on your shoulder." In a flash Monk A replied, "Brother, I saw a human being in need and did what was necessary. When I had carried the girl over the stream, I had done with her and could put her down. But look at you! You have carried her for seven miles!" (p. 129)

In the Japanese tradition the disciplines of work, family, and other social duties serve as the framework for both early and later development. Such mastery teaches acceptance and humility, and that notion is expressed by suffixing the term meaning "way" or "path" to the names of traditional pursuits (the way of tea, the way of fencing). To cultivate a particular way means to spend a long time practicing that art, deepening one's intuitive grasp of its nature. This concept has roots in both Chinese and Japanese philosophy. The peculiarly Japanese manifestation involves a conspicuous interplay between the discipline and mastery of work and the spiritual development of the individual. By virtue of the quality of attention one gives to even the most ordinary of tasks, living is raised to an art and all roles and duties are potentially of equal importance. Perseverance is valued highly, and abandoning one pursuit for another is viewed as debilitating and an indication of character weakness or immaturity. An individual who does not learn to concentrate and will not invest time and practice enough to gain insight and deeper understanding, whatever the undertaking, is likely to experience time as working against him and fail to achieve by his life's end the integrity that allows a dignified acceptance of his last season.

As it is for the Confucians, cultivation of the body as well as the mind is important to Japanese teachers. States of inner calm and stability are learned by practicing various forms of yoga. Calming the body enhances receptivity to outer reality and prepares one well for action. Here too the arts, from flower arranging to judo, involve the body continually, and diligence leads gradually to greater concentration, awareness, and equanimity.

Finally, with old age, the individual should transcend purely social forms and become more directly responsive to personal reality. Zen priests view personal growth as having come full circle when one achieves a final integrity comparable to the spontaneity and directness of a child (Rohlen, 1978). At the core of Japanese spiritualism is the example of the well-lived individual life.

THE ANCIENT GREEKS

A theme in the writings of the Greek philosophers that relates to the issues of development and maturation in the lives of individuals is that of activity vs. contemplation. The philosophical construct of contemplation as suitable to maturity was formulated to counteract the tyranny and injustice resulting from unchecked ambition and worldly glorification. In the active tradition, the ambitious politician, the tyrant, and the glory-seeking general are portrayed as self-centered, immature, and interested only in the ruthless enhancement of their own egos. By championing a contemplative, caring lifestyle, the Greek philosophers were proposing a new standard of adult maturity. Bellah (1978) uses Plato's parable of the cave to convey the essence of the new Platonic teaching about the ideal adult who is contemplative and cares for others.

> For the true contemplative man, who has left the cave to gaze on all things in the direct light of the sun, elects to return and to assist the dwellers in the cave, even unto the death. Guided by the vision of the heavenly city, which exists in the mode of eternity, the contemplative man *can act* for the welfare of the earthly city without being blinded by illusions of shining glory and immortal fame. (p. 66, italics added)

In the Socratic ideal, the philosopher is the properly educated man who escapes from the bonds of his senses to the freedom of enlightened reason and clear understanding of the realities of human existence. Only he is fit to govern, for he cares for the general welfare as well as that of individuals and will not be deterred from the pursuit of truth and justice by illusions of his own importance. Implicit in that ideal is the realization that a soul seeking "integrity and wholeness in all things human and divine" has a mind "habituated to thoughts of grandeur and the contemplation of all time and all existence," and that such a man "will not suppose death to be terrible" (Plato, *The Republic* Book VI). For the ancient Greek, as for his human counterparts in all previous and subsequent times, coming to terms with personal death is a central task of the mature adult.

CHRISTIANITY

Bouwsma (1978) identifies in the Christian tradition the theme of lifelong development and growth toward "mature manhood, measured by nothing less than the full stature of Christ . . . no longer to be children, tossed by the waves and whirled about by every fresh gust of teaching" (St. Paul, Ephes. 4:14). Because the goal of perfection is unattainable, the practical emphasis for the Christian adult is on growth through the challenges and problems encountered in living. His adult life, as his childhood, is a time of temptation and an occasion for achieving a closer tie to God. His spiritual life is in a constant state of flux, leading to spiritual growth or stagnation. The capacity to venture, to risk, in order to grow is essential to Christian adulthood, and Bouwsma notes that refusal of that challenge is an important source of sin. In Eden, Adam's rejection of his creatureliness and of his own potential for genuine growth are reflected in his narcissistic attempt to gain instant divinity by eating the forbidden fruit. He is left fearful of the future and afraid to grow. The concepts of confession, repentance, and salvation can be understood as means to recover the capacity for growth. He who cannot acknowledge that he is uncertain and unrighteous and has lost hope in this world—who cannot shed his narcissistic pretensions—cannot replace his anxiety with faith and so be able again to face his future. A key concept of modern developmental theory is that healthy growth does not occur without conflict. Conflict is a nearly constant feature of human existence which may either further development or impede it.

As with the mainstreams of the other major religious and philosophic movements, it is important for the Christian to live well within rather than apart from the community. Society is the proper arena in which to exercise one's soul, and the Christian ideal of maturity is realized only through identification and involvement with other people.

This review, though cursory, is intended to suggest the breadth and universality of certain themes related to the adult human experience. The overriding theme was well expressed in a statement attributed to Henri Bergson: "To exist is to change; to change is to mature; to mature is to create oneself endlessly" (Poulet, 1956, p. 36).

REFERENCES

Aries, P. *Centuries of childhood: A social history of family life.* New York: W. W. Norton, 1962.

Bellah, R. N. The active life and the contemplative life. In E. H. Erikson (Ed.), *Adulthood.* New York: W. W. Norton, 1978, pp. 61–80.

Bouwsma, W. J. Christian adulthood. In E. H. Erikson (Ed.), *Adulthood.* New York: W. W. Norton, 1978, pp. 81–96.

Caudill, W., & Weinstein, H. Maternal care and infant behavior in Japan and America. *Psychiatry,* 1969, 32, 12.

Erikson, E. H. (Ed.). *Adulthood.* New York: W. W. Norton, 1978.

Jordan, W. D. Searching for adulthood in America. In E. H. Erikson (Ed.), *Adulthood.* New York: W. W. Norton, 1978.

Levinson, D. J., Darrow, C. N., Klein, E. B., Levinson, M. H., & McKee, B. *The seasons of a man's life.* New York: Alfred A. Knopf, 1978.

Malia, M. E. Adulthood refracted: Russia and Leo Tolstoi. In E. H. Erikson (Ed.), *Adulthood.* New York: W. W. Norton, 1978.

Poulet, G. *[Studies in human time.]* (E. Coleman, trans.). Baltimore: Johns Hopkins University Press, 1956.

Rohlen, T. P. The promise of adulthood in Japanese spiritualism. In E. H. Erikson (Ed.), *Adulthood.* New York: W. W. Norton, 1978.

Shakespeare, W. *As you like it.* In G. B. Harrison (Ed.), *Shakespeare, the complete works.*
New York: Harcourt, Brace, 1952.
Tu, W. M. The Confucian perception of adulthood. In E. H. Erikson (Ed.), *Adulthood.*
New York: W. W. Norton, 1978.
vander Post, L. *A portrait of Japan.* New York: William Morrow, 1968.

2

The Pioneer Developmentalists

ARNOLD VAN GENNEP (1873–1957)

The first person to lay a foundation for the field of adult development was not a psychiatrist or psychoanalyst but an anthropologist. In 1908, Arnold Van Gennep originally published his monograph *The Rites of Passage* (Van Gennep, 1960), one of the first works to describe the importance and meaning of life events and rituals throughout the life span, making for his time a unique contribution to the social sciences. Examining the activities associated with such ceremonies in terms of their order and content, Van Gennep distinguished three major phases constituting the scheme of all rites of passage: *separation* from the group or society; *transition*, an intermediate learning stage; and *incorporation*, merger or return to the group in a new status or role. He commented upon the disturbances that changes in adult status produce in individuals, and saw rites of passage as social devices facilitating the reintegration of the individual with the group. Rites of passage help individuals with the critical tasks of becoming sexual beings, with changes in family or work relations, and with aging and death. With each life crisis these unique social rituals help an individual achieve his or her maximum potential and obtain group support in the adjustment.

Van Gennep classified and described, in a variety of cultural settings, rites associated with, among other events, pregnancy and childbirth, initiation, betrothal and marriage, death and funerals. The fact that his source of data ranged from the Australian bush to the communities of Europe emphasizes the universality of rites of passage (and, by implication, of development as well). His own words perhaps best summarize this conclusion:

The life of an individual in any society is a series of passages from one age to another and from one occupation to another. Whenever there are fine distinctions among age or occupational groups, progression from one group to the next is accompanied by special acts, like those which make up apprenticeship in our trades. Among semi-civilized peoples such acts are enveloped in ceremonies, since to the semi-civilized mind no act is entirely free of the sacred. In such societies every change in a person's life involves actions and reactions between sacred and profane—actions and reactions to be regulated and guarded so that society as a whole will suffer no discomfort or injury. Transitions from group to group and from one social situation to the next are looked on as implicit in the very fact of existence, so that a man's life comes to be made up of a succession of stages with similar ends and beginnings: birth, social puberty, marriage, fatherhood, advancement to a higher class, occupational specialization, and death. For every one of these events there are ceremonies whose essential purpose is to enable the individual to pass from one defined position to another which is equally well defined. (pp. 2–3)

In his introduction to Van Gennep's monograph, Kimball notes that the development of our urban, industrial civilization has produced increased secularization and a decline in sacred ceremonialism. In the past, rites of passage were frequently tied to supernatural sanctions and carried out by priestly intermediaries. Although the rites focused on the individual, they were also important occasions for group participation and community expression. There is little if any evidence that our secularized urban world has less need for ritualized expression of an individual's transition from one status to another; in fact, some contemporary social scientists and clinicians suggest that emotional problems may occur when individuals are forced to accomplish their transitions through life crises essentially alone, with private symbols and without the benefit of group sanction and support. To illustrate the importance of such prescribed activities for the individual and the group, we include here certain of Van Gennep's descriptions of key rites of passage.

Pregnancy and Childbirth

Of all the rites of passage, those of pregnancy and childbirth have been subject to the closest study. Attention has been drawn especially to customs of secluding the woman from the community. Pregnancy taboos are usually dietary and sexual. The woman is isolated either because she is considered impure and dangerous or because her condition is viewed as physiologically and/or socially abnormal. In many cultures nothing seems more natural than to treat the woman as if she were ill or a stranger.

In analyzing specific rites surrounding pregnancy and childbirth across many cultures, Van Gennep convincingly demonstrated the *universal* schema of *separation* of the woman from her usual environment and routine, followed by an extended state of *transition*, and finally by *reintegration* into the community life. Frequently this complex psychological-biological-social transition is divided into stages corresponding to the months considered important in the pregnancy—that is the third, fifth, seventh, eighth, and ninth months. The return to ordinary life is rarely made all at once; in many societies return is accomplished in stages that are similar to earlier initiation steps. Moreover, the transitional period usually continues beyond the time of delivery, although its duration varies among different peoples.

Van Gennep's description of the customs of the Hopi Indians of Oraibi, Arizona touches on several of these cross-cultural themes:

> As a rule, her mother is present during labor, and the woman remains at home; but neither her mother, her husband, her children, nor anyone else may be present at the delivery itself. When the child has arrived, her mother returns to assist, if necessary, in the expulsion of the placenta and to bind the baby's umbilical cord. Then her mother places on an old tray the placenta, pads, sand from under the woman, and the little broom, and carries it all to one of the placenta hills . . . of which there are several in close proximity to the village.
>
> For twenty days the young mother is subject to dietary taboos, and if it has been her first pregnancy she may not leave her house before sundown during this time, although she may do so after the fifth day if she has borne other children. On the fifth, tenth, and fifteenth days there is a ritual washing of both mother's and child's head and body; on the twentieth day the woman, her child, her mother, her husband, and other relatives are washed in this manner. On that day the women of the clan name the child, which is presented to the sun. Then all the family and the women who have named the child partake of a meal to which all the inhabitants of the pueblo are invited by the maternal grandmother, or even by a special crier. From that day on everything in the house goes its usual way for the mother, the child, the family, and the pueblo. (pp. 43–44)

The rites of pregnancy and childbirth differ in content from culture to culture, but are invariably comprised of processes of separation, transition, and reintegration. Almost all include a passage over or across something, joint prayers, and symbolic or real sacrifices. Designated people play the roles of intermediaries. The ceremonies are intended not only to neutralize impurities or evil sorcery (i.e., facilitate delivery and protect mother and child, and sometimes father, close relatives, and the whole family or clan, against misfortune), but "to serve as actual bridges, chains, or links—in short, to facilitate the changing condition without violent social disruptions or an abrupt cessation of individual and collective life" (p. 48). From the complexity of the processes involved and the intensity of the human experience, it is clear such rites have considerable individual and social impact on the formation of the adult self and the course of adult development.

Initiation Rites

Initiation rites per se are crucial to the assumption of adult status in most societies. Van Gennep noted that physiological puberty and social puberty are essentially different and rarely converge, and, indeed, in Western society the gap between them seems to be ever widening. He described initiation ceremonies of all sorts, including those that bring about admission to certain age groups or secret societies, accompany the ordination of a priest or shaman, mark the enthroning of a king, or celebrate the consecration of monks and nuns or sacred prostitutes.

As an example, some of the most dramatic initiation rites occur when a boy passes into manhood, often by initiation into a totem group. Such ceremonies have been studied across cultures in minute detail. They may last for a considerable length of time, extending in some groups over years. The sequence always begins with a separation from the previous environment, including the world of women and children. The man-to-be is secluded in a special place, and his behavior is subject to many taboos, frequently of a dietary nature. The boy's link with his mother may endure for some time, but a moment always comes when they are finally separated from each other, often abruptly if not violently. It is striking that in some tribes during the initiation period the novice is considered dead. The rationale behind the practice is to make him lose all recollection of childhood. Then he is instructed in tribal law, hears recitations of myths, witnesses totem ceremonies, and undergoes some special mutilation (e.g., removal of a tooth or incision of the penis) which renders him identical with all other adult males in the tribe. Thus the schema holds: The novice is considered dead (separation from childhood past); is resurrected and taught how to live differently than as a child (transition); and undergoes a change symbolizing identification and acceptance as an adult (reintegration). The rites of passage into manhood in some societies are undergone simultaneously by a group of initiates. In a sense the passage is a double one—separation from the usual environment; incorporation into a sacred environment; a transitional period; then separation from the sacred environment followed by reincorporation into the usual one.

Initiation rites, of course, do not occur only at the passage from adolescence to adulthood, for changes of status throughout the life cycle are accompanied by rituals. Van Gennep described initiation ceremonies for the priesthood or shamanism among various peoples. Such procedures are particularly interesting because they extend well into the adult years, and exemplify the dynamic process of change in adulthood. In form and process, if not in content, they might be compared to the successive stages of training and certification undergone in contemporary Western society by individuals entering certain professions or lines of work such as medicine or the skilled trades. An example of the elaborate complexity involved in such social processes appears in Van Gennep's description of the process to which candidates for the priesthood are subject among the Sabians of Iraq.

> Baptism plays an important part in their ascension from one ecclesiastical grade to another and in all the life of the novices, deacons, priests, and bishops. A novice must be a legitimate son of a priest or bishop, and he must be without physical defect; if he is judged worthy after an examination, he receives a special baptism, studies from seven to nineteen years, and is then ordained deacon. At the end of six months or a year as a deacon, if an assembly of the people wish it, he is ordained a priest. He is confined in a reed hut; for seven days and seven nights he must not soil himself and may not sleep. Each day he changes his clothes and must give alms. On the eighth day a funeral is held for him, since he is considered dead. Afterwards he is accompanied by four priests to the river, where they administer baptism to him. During the sixty days that follow he bathes himself three times a day, and if he has a nocturnal emission that day does not count among the sixty. The days on which either his mother or his wife have menses are not counted, so that it sometimes takes four or five months to accumulate sixty days free of all pollution. (p. 107)

Betrothal and Marriage

The rites surrounding betrothal and marriage are especially significant because in many cultures marriage constitutes the most important adult transition from one social category to another. For at least one of the spouses it usually involves a change of family, clan, village, or tribe. With the newly married couple establishing residence in a new place, there are many rituals of separation, primarily focused on territorial passage. Van Gennep described the elaborate betrothal rites of the Bhotiya, who live in southern Tibet and Sikkim. After astrologers have determined whether signs for the union are auspicious, the couples' uncles, acting as go-betweens, meet in the boy's home and then take gifts to the girl's family and ask for her in marriage. Upon acceptance of the gifts the dowry is agreed upon, whereupon the uncles are given a feast, and there are prayers to bless the bride and groom. After those rites of familial incorporation the couple may meet in complete freedom. A year later the groom's parents host a meal for all the relatives, and the bride is paid for at that time. After another year, the astrologer indicates a favorable date for the bride to leave her parents' home, and details are decided in light of his suggestions. A great celebration is planned, to which the lamas (priests or monks of Mahayana Buddhism) are invited. During the celebration two men enact a simulated abduction of the bride. The "thieves" are spared a beating and have half-cooked meat thrown into their mouths if they give money to the bride's guardians. (Two days later they will be honored as "the happy strategists.") The bride and her parents receive gifts from their guests, and all depart in joyous procession toward the groom's home. They are met en route and escorted the rest of the way by his parents. After two or three days of celebration the girl and her parents return to their home. Another year passes before the bride's dowry is given (double the amount paid for her) and then she is escorted to her husband's home, to remain permanently.

Death and Funeral Rites

The death of an individual and its effect on the living give rise to complex and meaningful rites of passage in all cultures. Although the expectation might be that for the dead the rites of separation would be the most prominent, and rites of transition and incorporation less so, that is not the case. Rites of separation are generally few in number and very simple, whereas ceremonies of transition and incorporation of the deceased into the world of the dead are more elaborate and significant.

Likewise, survivors enter a transitional process of mourning through rites of separation, and upon emergence are reintegrated with the community of the living. As Van Gennep stated,

> during mourning, the living mourners and the deceased constitute a special group, situated between the world of the living and the world of the dead, and how soon living individuals leave that group depends on the closeness of their relationship with the dead person. (p. 147)

As we have seen, death, transitional states between this world and the afterworld, and rites of resurrection also play a part in many of the ceremonies of pregnancy, childbirth, initiation, betrothal, and marriage. In Chapter 1 we stressed the central roles that the meaning of mortality seemed to have in the great religions and cultures of the world. Thus among primitive and civilized peoples, anxiety about death and the need to integrate its personal and societal meanings play central roles in the everyday ceremonies and rites of passage that make up the individual and societal life cycle. It is almost as if the mastery of that anxiety were fostered by the culture's insitutions to facilitate the integration of both the individual and the community.

SIGMUND FREUD (1856–1939)

Psychoanalysis offered the first modern, systematic theory of personality development, and Freud's main developmental ideas have formed the basis for much subsequent theoretical work. Before Freud, theorists conceived of growth and development essentially as the unwinding of hidden springs within the organism. His genius brought together biology and psychology, describing development as the *interaction* between forces within the organism (biological constitution) and forces in the environment (life's psychological experiences), emphasizing not only the interaction of biological and psychological variables, but the basic *interdependence* of organism and environment.

The fundamental hypotheses of psychoanalytic developmental psychology were described as early as 1905 in Freud's pioneering monograph, *Three Essays on the Theory of Sexuality*. Recently Abrams (1978) has summarized these as follows:

> 1. Maturational emergence: There is an expected sequence of emerging functions in the psychic apparatus leading to progressively differentiated structures of hierarchical organization; the sequence, the functions, and the structures are rooted in biological sources.

2. Milieu: To materialize and flourish, each requires environmental stimulation. The range of stimulation and the timing are important variables influencing outcome.

3. Experiential interface: The experiential products of the "outer" and "inner" interaction also codetermine what is to follow.

4. Transformations: Each step in the sequence involves transformations as well as sequences.

5. Progression-regression processes: Development is also effected by intrinsic regressive and progressive processes which influence intensity, duration, and cadence. (pp. 388–389)

Abrams describes Freud's elaboration of the five hypotheses. "Maturational emergence" is illustrated by the libido theory, the emergence of oral, anal, and phallic drives as a biological developmental sequence. "Milieu" refers to the types of environmental stimuli available to effect and respond to the oral, anal, and phallic manifestations. "Experiential interface" describes the role of frustration and excessive gratification in the development of fixations at any stage, and their critical impact on later development. "Transformations" appear in the concept of sublimation of sexual aims. "Progression–regression processes" are represented by shifts, arrests, or fixations in the range of developmental phenomena.

From the standpoint of developmental theory, Freud's ideas of psychosexual genesis were the beginning of a psychodynamic understanding of development. There are both "push" and "pull" in development. For the individual, factors of physiological and psychological maturation provide stimuli and "push," but there is a tendency to maintain the status quo at any given stage, giving rise to a "pull" back toward already achieved levels of development. When comfortable and satisfied we are inclined not to strive for new forms of independence. Freud was the first to examine systematically how we react to the process of being "weaned" in the oral, anal, and phallic stages from the mother and by the mother. He and his colleagues divided that developmental process into five relatively separate but temporally overlapping stages:

- The oral stage, further subdivided into oral sucking and oral biting. Weaning from the breast or bottle is the main frustration of the child.
- The anal stage, subdivided into anal expulsive and anal retentive. Frustration in this stage has to do with issues of toilet training.

- The phallic stage. The chief frustrations in this stage have to do with infantile masturbation and possession of the parent of the opposite sex.
- The latency period, during which the experience of psychosexuality is largely repressed.
- The genital stage in which, with puberty, there is a reemergence of psychosexuality.

Information about the psychosexual stages of development as understood by the *early* psychoanalysts has been well tabulated by Brown (1940) (see Table I).

Freud did not pay much attention to the adult years as a series of further developmental stages. He described maturity as the ability to work and love, but, perhaps because of the great significance of his discoveries about childhood, he devoted himself to elucidating the impact of those early interpersonal experiences on later mental life. His description of the persistence of infantile and childhood themes in both the conscious and unconscious content of adult experience and behavior has led to the charge that he and the other early psychoanalysts were excessively reductionistic in their descriptions of adult personality. Although it is true that in the main Freud neglected the adult years, he did have some understanding of the ways individuals continue to change and grow throughout life. Consider the advice he gave to psychoanalysts in one of his last papers,

> Every analyst should periodically—at intervals of five years or so—submit himself to analysis once more, without feeling ashamed of taking this step. This would mean, then, that not only the therapeutic analysis of patients, but his own analysis would change from a terminable into an interminable task. (Freud, 1937, p. 249)

CARL GUSTAV JUNG (1875–1961)

Perhaps it is not widely appreciated that Carl Jung, originally a disciple of Freud and a leading member of the early psychoanalytic movement, was the first psychoanalyst to write profoundly and extensively about the second half of life. He felt that young adults in their twenties and thirties were involved in both freeing themselves of their childhood conflicts and trying to establish themselves with new families and careers. He believed, moreover, that a significant opportunity for psychological change and growth occurred around age forty. Call-

TABLE I. *Psychosexual*

Name	Age	Libidinal localization	Libidinal mode	Libidinal object	Theoretical normal development		
					Frustration conflict	Complex	Behavioral results
1	2	3	4	5	6	7	8
Oral sucking	Birth to 8 mos.	Mouth, lips, tongue	Sucking, swallowing Introjection Preambivalent	Autoerotic Passive, dependent	Weaning	Beginnings of Oedipus complex Mother choice of both sexes	Development of oral aggressiveness Ambivalence
Oral biting	6 to 18 mos.	Teeth, jaws	Biting, devouring, destroying Sadistic introjection Ambivalent	Autoerotic and narcissistic Oral-sadistic attachment to mother	Final weaning New child	Continuation of ambivalent Oedipus complex Mother choice of both sexes	First consciousness of reality Feeling of being cheated Anal interest
Anal expulsive	8 mos. to 3 yrs.	Anus and buttocks	Expelling, rejecting, destroying Projection Ambivalent	Continued narcissism and anal attachment to parents	Necessity of sphincter control	Continuation of ambivalent Oedipus complex Realization of sexuality Both sexes conscious of father	Social reality Feeling of power Development of sphincter control
Anal retentive	12 mos. to 4 yrs.	Anus, buttocks, sphincter control Urethra	Retaining and controlling feces and urine Ambivalent	Continued narcissistic and anal-sadistic attachment to both parents	Need to accept social reality and complete sphincter control	Castration in girl Beginnings of positive Oedipus in boy	Development of interest in genitalia
Phallic	3 to 7 yrs.	Urethra and outer genitalia Clitoris and penis	Urinating Infantile masturbation Ambivalent	Oedipus choice on ambivalent level	Threat of castration for infantile masturbation	Castration in boy and renunciation in girl	Repression of infantile sexuality
Latency	5 to 12 yrs.	No new zone Old zones denied	Repression and reaction formation	Decline of autoeroticism and development of social feelings	Behavioral problems of late childhood	Superego conflicts of late childhood	"Boy and girl scout" behavior
Genital	12 to 20 yrs.	Genitalia	Coitus Postambivalence	First homosexual crushes, hero worship, then heterosexual sex objects	Puberty	Adolescent homosexuality	Adolescent masturbation Interest in opposite sex

[a] From Brown, 1940, pp. 204–206 ("combined with some modification from the similar ones of Abraham (1927), Healy, Bronner, and Bowers, Rickman (1928a), and an unpublished table of W. C. Menninger").

Stages of Development[a]

Structural results	Normal behavior formation			Symptom formation		
	Continuations	Sublimations	Reaction formations	Psychosis or neurosis	Perversion	Character defect
9	10	11	12	13	14	15
Pleasure principle overwhelmingly predominant Practically all id and unconscious	Drinking Eating (chewing) Smoking Kissing Oral hygiene, etc.	Wine tasting Epicureanism Oratory Wit Sarcasm, etc.	Food faddism Dislike of milk Prohibition enthusiasm Purism in speech Continual visiting of dentists, etc.	Schizophrenia Manic-depressive	Passive oral-inversion Active oral-sadism	Schizoid Narcissistic Infantile Cycloid?
First development of reality sense; emergence of ego and conscious						
Reality of growing importance Ego definitely developed Beginnings of superego (level of reality testing)	Interest in daily bowel movement Constipation, diarrhea Erotic pleasure in defecation "Chic Sale literature," anal stories, etc.	Painting Sculpture Philanthropy Statistical studies, etc.	Disgust with feces Excessive fear of dirt Prudishness Pedantry Parsimony Petulance, etc.	Paranoia Compulsion neurosis	Passive anal-inversion Homosexuality Active anal-sadism	Paranoid Compulsive
Reality overbears pleasure Ego development essentially complete Beginnings of identification and superego	Masturbation Narcissistic dating Petting Dirty jokes Dancing, etc.	Love poetry Acting Sacred love, etc.	Puritanism regarding sex Modesty, etc.	Anxiety hysteria Conversion hysteria	Phallic narcissism Exhibitionism, voyeurism Nymphomania Satyrisis	Neurotic Hysterical
Reality established Superego complete Id repressed into conscious	The continuations, sublimations, and reaction formations of the latency period include all the others in a socially modified form.					
Establishment of superego						
Reemergence of pleasure principle and id drives Personality complete	Normal sex life	Renunciation of sex for art, science, society Rejection of sexuality	Socially constructive work	At the genital level there are no symptoms found		

ing forty "the noon of life," he described continued personality individuation during the second half of the life cycle. In one of the first
psychological descriptions of midlife transitions, Jung (1933) wrote:

> Experience shows us rather that the basis and cause of all the difficul-
> ties of this transition are to be found in a deep-seated and peculiar change
> within the psyche. In order to characterize it I must take for comparison the
> daily course of the sun—but a sun that is endowed with human feeling and
> man's limited consciousness. In the morning it arises from the nocturnal sea
> of unconsciousness and looks upon the wide, bright world which lies be-
> fore it in an expanse that steadily widens the higher it climbs in the firma-
> ment. In this extension of its field of action caused by its own rising, the
> sun will discover its significance; it will see the attainment of the greatest
> possible height—the widest possible dissemination of its blessing—as its
> goal. In this conviction the sun pursues its unforeseen course to the zenith;
> unforeseen, because its career is unique and individual, and its culminating
> point could not be calculated in advance. At the stroke of noon the descent
> begins. And the descent means the reversal of all the ideals and values that
> were cherished in the morning. The sun falls into contradiction with itself.
> It is as though it should draw in its rays, instead of emitting them. Light
> and warmth decline and are at last extinguished. (p. 106)

Jung felt that until the "zenith," important aspects of a man's or
woman's self were neglected or suppressed. During mid-adulthood
significant features of thought, feeling, intuition, and sensation could
be further developed and integrated. As an example, he described how
men during their forties seem to become more aware of their feminine
sides and women seem to become more comfortable with the masculine aspects of their personalities.

> How often it happens that a man of forty or fifty years winds up his
> business, and that his wife then dons the trousers and opens a little shop
> where he sometimes performs the duties of handyman. There are many
> women who only awake to social responsibility and to social consciousness
> after their fortieth year. In modern business life—especially in the United
> States—nervous breakdown in the forties or after is a very common occur-
> rence. If one studies the victims a little closely one sees that the thing which
> has broken down is the masculine style of life which held the field up to
> now; what is left over is an effeminate man. Contrariwise, one can observe
> women in these self-same business spheres who have developed in the sec-
> ond half of life an uncommon masculinity and an incisiveness which push
> the feelings and the heart aside. Very often the reversal is accompanied by
> all sorts of catastrophes in marriage; for it is not hard to imagine what may
> happen when the husband discovers his tender feelings, and the wife her
> sharpness of mind. (pp. 107–108)

Another important contribution of Jung to the understanding of
adult development is that of the archetype "Puer," or Young, and the

archetype "Senex," or Old. In Jungian theory an archetype is an elemental unconscious image that has been established over thousands of generations in human evolution. The archetypes evolve in an individual mind from an initial, undifferentiated image into more and more complex images. Levinson, Darrow, Klein, Levinson, and McKee (1978) believe that in every transitional period, throughout the life cycle, Jung's archetypes Puer and Senex are modified, reintegrated, and put in new balance. He describes Puer and Senex as a fundamental polarity in each stage of life.

In summary, Jung saw development as continuous throughout the life cycle and expressed the idea that the serious problems of life are never fully solved. He felt that the challenge of a problem did not rest in its solution, but in our working at it incessantly, which "alone preserves us from stultification and petrification" (p. 103). In a semiserious vein Jung pointed out that adults are wholly unprepared for the second half of life and wished for colleges for forty-year olds to prepare them for the second half of life and its demands, as the ordinary college introduces young people to the adult world.

Erik H. Erikson (born 1902)

Whereas Freud in creating psychoanalysis initiated the modern study of human development, and Jung was the first psychoanalyst to give particular attention to the adult years, Erik Erikson, a child psychoanalyst, provided the first psychosocially integrated view of how an individual develops *throughout* the life cycle. Erikson has had enormous influence in various fields, including psychology, psychoanalysis, the social sciences, and the humanities. His most influential book is *Childhood and Society (1963)*, which contains his original delineation of the eight stages of life. Since writing it he has devoted himself to understanding adult development, uniquely combining psychoanalytical, biographical, and historical-sociological modes of study. This enterprise has produced a series of books, each of which has both illuminated its particular subject and, perhaps even more importantly, pioneered methodology for the study of adult development and psychohistory: *Young Man Luther* (1958), *Insight and Responsibility* (1964), *Identity— Youth and Crisis* (1968), *On the Origins of Militant Nonviolence* (1969), *In Search of Common Ground* (with Huey P. Newton and Kai T. Erikson, 1973a), and *Dimensions of a New Identity: Jefferson Lectures* (1973b).

Building initially on the work of Freud, Anna Freud (his first psychoanalytic mentor), and other early psychoanalysts, Erikson extended the view that development grows out of the interaction of both internal (psychological) and external (social) events. The foundation of development lies in change rather than stability. As an individual progresses through life he or she is confronted with contradiction, conflict, and disequilibrium. Central to Erikson's view of development is the "epigenetic" principle, which states that anything that grows has an internal "game plan." Embryologists have demonstrated that in fetal development each aspect has a critical time of ascendancy and corresponding vulnerability to distortion (Erikson, 1959). This is not a static description because at each stage of life a new strength is "added to a widening ensemble and re-integrated at each later stage in order to play its part in a full cycle . . . " (1969, p. 38). Finally, order and development do not occur randomly. Growth takes place step-by-step and at a predictable rate and sequence. As Erikson writes, "Steps must not only be fitted to each other, they must also add up to a definite direction and perspective" (1966, p. 618).

Erikson denies that the epigenetic view characterizes development as a series of negative crises. He claims only that "psychosocial development proceeds by critical steps—'critical' being a characteristic of turning points, of moments of decision between progress and regression, integration and retardation" (1963, pp. 270–271). He further feels that each stage in the life cycle implies potential growth since

> Developmental and normative crises differ from imposed, traumatic, and neurotic crises in that the very process of growth provides new energy even as society offers new and specific opportunities according to its dominant conception of the phases of life. (1968, pp. 162–163)

Each of Erikson's stages is organized around a crucial developmental issue for the individual self in relation to the social world. The issue is described as a polarity—two seeming opposites between which exists a creative tension that results for each individual in a unique mixture or blend of the feelings (Figure 1).

The first stage, from birth to two years, is analogous to what Freud called the oral stage. Erikson calls it the incorporative stage. The *basic trust* and *mistrust* developed during that period constitute the source of "both primal hope and of doom throughout life" (1963, p. 80). This sense of trust grows from the relative certainty of comfort and constancy when the parent provides consistency, continuity, and a basic

	1	2	3	4	5	6	7	8
VIII MATURITY								EGO INTEGRITY VS. DESPAIR
VII ADULTHOOD							GENERA-TIVITY VS. STAGNATION	
VI YOUNG ADULTHOOD						INTIMACY VS. ISOLATION		
V PUBERTY AND ADOLESCENCE					IDENTITY VS. ROLE CONFUSION			
IV LATENCY				INDUSTRY VS. INFERIORITY				
III LOCOMOTOR-GENITAL			INITIATIVE VS. GUILT					
II MUSCULAR-ANAL		AUTONOMY VS. SHAME, DOUBT						
I ORAL SENSORY	BASIC TRUST VS. MISTRUST							

FIGURE 1. The stages of human development and corresponding developmental issues for the individual self.

responsiveness to the very young child's needs. The very earliest sense that one can rely on another person's integrity is related to faith on the infant's part in the mother and is the first building block in the evolution of interpersonal relations. In contrast, Erikson found that psychotic individuals had early child-rearing situations that engendered considerable mistrust via unpredictable and chaotic parenting:

> We could speak here of a psychosocial weakness which consists of a readiness to mistrust and to lose hope in rather fundamental ways . . . . Frieda Fromm-Reichman was a doctor who doggedly sat down with psychotics as if saying,"I'm not going to give up until you trust again."(Evans, 1967, p. 55)

The second stage, two to four years, has as its center conflict *autonomy vs. shame and doubt,* and corresponds to the anal stage in Freudian terms. However, Erikson broadens the familiar conflicts over toilet training to the need of the child to develop his or her first sense of psychosocial independence or autonomy. As the child struggles with toilet training and taking the first symbolic steps away from parents, shame can develop if instances of failure are not handled sensitively. Shame can produce deviousness or defiance because the child may develop a fear of being discovered or stared at. Doubt seems to occur when the child experiences repeated failure, and the balance between self-control and self-expression is lost. Erikson feels that resolution of the conflict between autonomy and shame or doubt is all-important for the eventual development of love and hate. Further, "if in some respects you have relatively more shame than autonomy then you feel or act inferior all your life—or consistently counteract that feeling" (Evans, 1967, p. 31). To state the resolution of the polarity between autonomy and shame or doubt in a different way,

> from a sense of self control without loss of self esteem comes a lasting sense of autonomy and pride; from a sense of muscular and anal impotence, a loss of self control, and of parental overcontrol comes a lasting sense of doubt and shame. (Erikson, 1968, p. 113)

The third stage, four to seven years, is characterized by a conflict over *initiative* vs. *guilt*, corresponding to the oedipal stage, when the child is beginning a "generational battle" with his parents. Because the child wants the prerogatives of the same-sex parent, including the sole possession of the opposite-sex parent, he or she experiments with taking initiative in a variety of ways. The danger is that if the child takes or is given more responsibility than he can handle, significant guilt may arise. During this stage the early development of the child's superego is most obvious. Self-observation, self-guidance, and self-punishment develop as parental prohibitions are internalized and become part of the self.

The fourth stage, seven to 12 years, corresponds to the time referred to by Freud as "latency," wherein the conflict is expressed as *industry* vs. *inadequacy*. This is the school age for most children, the time when they develop a sense of competence as they begin to develop the skills of work. Along with industriousness come the social skills of being able to get along with others. The danger is that feelings of inadequacy may grow in the child who does not learn easily and well.

In the fifth stage, adolescence, Erikson has contributed a major idea to psychology by describing how personal identity is developed through the interaction of *identity* vs. *role confusion*. The adolescent strives to create a coherent and integrated sense of self by physically and psychologically separating from parents. During this span of ages, 12 to 20, the adolescent may experience considerable "identity diffusion," that is, feeling lost, confused, alienated, and unmotivated to invest the self. As he resolves confusion over the changes in his body and his relations to peers and parents, a new sense of identity emerges.

In his sixth, seventh, and eighth stages Erikson takes psychology and psychiatry beyond a constricted view of the life cycle to a more comprehensive view of development as lifelong. Here for the first time is an organized scheme for the description and study of development during the adult years. During the sixth or young-adult stage (twenties and thirties), individuals struggle with issues of *intimacy* vs. *self-absorption*. As in each of the above stages, how one has resolved the preceding crisis plays an important part, and that resolution is particularly critical for the achievement of intimacy. Intimacy, according to Erikson, includes sexual relating; but is more than sexual and has to do with caring and sharing as well. True intimacy requires that one experience someone else's needs and concerns as equally important to one's own. To have genuine concern for another, one needs a cohesive sense of personal self and relatively little fear or anxiety about losing oneself in giving to another, whether it be on the intellectual, emotional, or sexual plane. Intimacy requires near fusion of one's identity with that of another, and to achieve that, in sexual relations or in marriage, one must be able to face the threat of ego loss. If one cannot, one faces the dangers of *isolation* and *self-absorption*.

The sense of isolation comes into particular prominence in young adulthood when an individual's social options may have narrowed and the support of school or the adolescent peer group is no longer present. A young adult must take initiatives in engaging others. If inferiority and role confusion predominate, friendships are difficult to establish, intimacy does not develop, and loneliness and alienation can establish a pattern of isolation and self-absorption. The recluse is, of course, the extreme, but there are many shades of self-absorption, including people who live and work among but not really with other people.

During the seventh stage (forties and fifties), or the "midlife period," the conflict between *generativity* and *stagnation* emerges. For Erikson successful generativity, the care and facilitation of a younger generation, is the key to fulfillment and cohesion in middle age. That idea seems alien to the contemporary narcissistic emphasis on exclusive self-fulfillment, "the me generation." However, in the usual course of events the outcome of the young-adult struggle with intimacy vs. isolation is marriage and the establishment of a family. Boundless opportunities for generativity occur in rearing children and participating in programs for youth. Erikson believes that adults *need* children, and that they need to take care of someone just as children need to be cared for. Adults in their forties and fifties learn how to guide the next generation through their parenting, teaching, creativity, and participation in society. Our social institutions of adult life, including marriage, parenthood, and work, require the development of the ability to be generative and in turn guarantee generative succession. Of course marriage and children are not the only means to developing a sense of generativity. Many activities allow single people opportunities to work with and for others. Furthermore, having a family does not automatically promote generative abilities; for some parents children are a threat to fragile selves.

Individuals who are not able to be generative feel a sense of personal stagnation. In despair, they feel stuck, as if they are standing still intellectually and emotionally. Such feelings give rise to intense midlife evaluations from which some individuals move in positive new directions, while others flounder. Willy Loman in Arthur Miller's *Death of a Salesman* or Scrooge in Charles Dickens's *A Christmas Carol* are both men who seem to have lost any sense of forward momentum and are involved in a self-centered, materialistic, here-and-now existence. In both of these stories the characters emerge from their stagnation, for a while, when they are able to be concerned for the young.

According to Erikson, the eighth and final stage in the life cycle (the sixties and beyond) brings either a sense of *integrity* or a sense of *despair*. As individuals enter the last phase of their lives, they reflect upon their time and how it has been lived. When one has taken care of things and people relatively successfully and adapted to the triumphs and disappointments, one can look back with mostly satisfaction and only a few regrets: one experiences a sense of integrity about oneself, feeling that one has lived totally and well and one's life has been meaningful. Integrity of the self allows one to accept inevitable disease and death without fear of succumbing helplessly. However, if an individual looks back on his or her life as a series of missed opportunities, or as filled with personal misfortune, the sense is one of bitter despair, a preoccupation about what might have been "if only" this or that had happened. Then death is fearsome, for it symbolizes emptiness.

One of Erikson's most important contributions has been to make explicit the processes inherent in each stage of human growth which offer the potential for fresh personal strength to overcome older weaknesses of the self. The most succinct notion of the promise of lifelong development was expressed when he closed a lecture series as follows:

> . . . but now I have only one minute left to indicate what an adult is. . . . From the point of view of development, I would say: In youth you find out what you *care to do* and who you *care to be*—even in changing roles. In young adulthood you learn whom you *care to be with*—at work and in private life, not only exchanging intimacies but sharing intimacy. In adulthood, however, you learn to know what and whom you can *take care of*. I have said all of this in basic American before; but I must add that as a principle it corresponds to what in Hinduism is called the maintenance of the world, that middle period of the life cycle when existence permits you and demands you to consider death as peripheral and to balance its certainty with the only happiness that is lasting: to increase, by whatever is yours to give, the good will and the higher order in your sector of the world. That to me, can be the only adult meaning of that strange word *happiness* as a political principle. (1973b, p. 124)

REFERENCES

Abrams, S. The teaching and learning of psychoanalytic developmental psychology. *Journal of the American Psychoanalytic Association, 1978, 26,* 387.

Brown, J. F. *The psychodynamics of abnormal behavior.* New York: McGraw-Hill, 1940.

Erikson, E. H. *Young man Luther.* New York: W. W. Norton, 1958.

Erikson, E. H. *Identity and the life cycle: Selected papers.* New York: International Universities Press, 1959.

Erikson, E. H. *Childhood and society* (2nd ed.). New York: W. W. Norton, 1963.

Erikson, E. H. *Insight and responsibility: Lectures on the ethical implications of psychoanalytic insight.* New York: W. W. Norton, 1964.

Erikson, E. H. The ontogeny of ritualization. In R. Lowenstein, L. Newman, M. Shur, & A. Solnit (Eds.), *Psychoanalysis, a general psychology: Essays in honor of Heinz Hartmann.* New York: International Universities Press, 1966, pp. 601–621.

Erikson, E. H. *Identity—youth and crisis.* New York: W. W. Norton, 1968.

Erikson, E. H. *Gandhi's truth: On the origins of militant nonviolence.* New York: W. W. Norton, 1969.

Erikson, E. H. *In search of common ground: Conversations with Erik H. Erikson and Huey P. Newton.* New York: W. W. Norton, 1973. (a)

Erikson, E. H. *Dimensions of a new identity: Jefferson lectures.* New York: W. W. Norton, 1973. (b)

Evans, R. I. *Dialogue with Erik Erikson.* New York: Harper & Row, 1967.

Freud, S. *Three essays on the theory of sexuality.* Standard edition 7:125. London: Hogarth Press, 1905.

Freud, S. *Analysis terminable and interminable.* Standard edition 23:216. London: Hogarth Press, 1937.

Jung, C. G. *Modern man in search of a soul.* New York: Harcourt, Brace, 1933.

Van Gennep, A. *The rites of passage.* (M. B. Vizedom & G. L. Caffee, trans.). Chicago: University of Chicago Press, 1960.

3

Contemporary Adult Developmentalists

Having discussed the life cycle and images of adulthood from the perspectives of some scholars of antiquity and pioneer developmentalists, we will now describe the thinking of contemporary researchers. The study of adult development is really in its infancy, especially when compared to our knowledge of childhood and adolescence. It is appropriate, we believe, to wonder why the study of the adult has lagged so far behind. Stevens-Long (1979) suggests that the attention paid to children and adolescents, as opposed to adults, has its roots in economic, social, and psychological issues. The spread of compulsory education, with large numbers of children attending public schools, forced educators and psychologists to conduct developmental studies to provide information about optimal teaching methods, classroom organization, discipline, and social behavior. Both biologists and psychologists stressed that the study of children was an important source of information about the evolution of the species. Freud's revolutionary description of early development and its effects in later life for a long time precluded very much attention being paid to exclusively adult facets of experience.

It probably makes sense to look at investigators themselves to understand the resistances involved in studying adult psychology. The people studying normal adult behavior are by and large middle-aged; to confront the data and ask the necessary questions means confronting themselves, and that may have provoked resistances only now being surmounted.

Stevens-Long (1979) suggests that perhaps the study of adult psychology had to wait for economic and social forces similar to those that focused attention on children. For instance, at the turn of the century the average life span for males was about 45 years; now many men and women can expect to live beyond 70. This change has made the study of the adult years or the "second half of life" considerably more relevant for social scientists as well as for society at large.

Neugarten (1979), surveying adult-developmental studies, points out that about 20 years ago gerontologists started to ask about the antecedents of *different* patterns of old age. Now they are focusing on the *process of aging* rather than *the aged*, leading to an extension of such studies *downward* in the life cycle. She further points out that child psychologists conducting longitudinal studies of infants and children found themselves following their study populations upward into adulthood: the two groups "joined up in the middle, and there is now a growing interest in the whole life cycle as a unit for study." To summarize the modern study of adult development we will present data that have appeared primarily in three major studies: *The Seasons of a Man's Life*, by Daniel Levinson and his associates at Yale (1978); *Adaptation to Life*, by George Vaillant of Harvard (1977); and *Transformations*, by Roger Gould of UCLA (1978). The important thinking of Bernice Neugarten, Robert Lifton, and George Pollock will also be noted.

DANIEL J. LEVINSON AND *THE SEASONS OF A MAN'S LIFE*

The most comprehensive and heuristic modern study of adult development has been carried out by Daniel Levinson and his associates and reported in their book *The Seasons of a Man's Life* (1978). They advance an empirically derived, psychosocial theory of adult development in which men progress through a series of life stages as they move from early into middle and late adulthood. Each stage and the transitions between them are demarked chronologically. Although the stages are broadly based on Erikson's stages of ego development, there are important differences. Levinson's group focused less on the changes occurring within the person and more on the interface between the self and the interpersonal world. Because their methods offer an important model for adult-developmental studies, we shall describe them briefly.

The research sample consisted of four groups of 10 each: biologists, novelists, business executives, and blue-collar workers, 40 men from 35 to 40 years old. The heart of their research method involved "biographical interviewing," from 10 to 20 hours of personal interviews with each person. Also, each individual was asked to respond to a selected series of pictures from the Murray Thematic Apperception Test. The primary task as explained to the subjects was for interviewer and interviewee to construct the story of the man's life. The research group tried to cover the entire life sequence from childhood to adulthood, including the family of origin; marriage and family of procreation; all important relationships with men and women; education; occupational choice and work history; leisure activities; involvement in ethnic, religious, political and other interests; illness; death and loss of loved ones; and turning points in the life course.

Thus the essential approach was to elicit the life stories of 40 men, to construct their biographies, and to develop generalizations based upon those biographies. In each case, the research group began by immersing themselves in the interview material and worked toward an intuitive understanding of its contents, in the process producing a systematic construction of the 40 life courses. In addition to the primary sample of 40 men, the lives of men as depicted in biographies, autobiographies, novels, plays, and poems were also studied.

Levinson's psychosocial theory of adult development proposes a universal life cycle consisting of specific eras and periods in a set sequence from birth to old age. The basic unit of the life cycle is the *era*, which lasts about 20 years; that is: preadulthood, 0–20, early adulthood, 20–40, middle adulthood, 40–60, late adulthood, 60–80, and late, late adulthood, 80 on. Each era has its distinctive character (Figure 2). Berman and Lief (1975) have correlated individual and marital stages of development in a useful application of the Levinson developmental periods (Table II).

The basic developmental process in adulthood is construed as the evolution of an individual *life structure*, "the underlying design of the person's life at a given time . . . a patterning of self-in-world [which] requires us to take into account both self and world" (Newton & Levinson, 1979, p. 488). The life structure is not static nor does it change in unpredictable ways; it evolves in a systematic, sequential *alternation* of stable and transitional periods. In a stable period, which usually lasts six or seven years, an individual is primarily building structure and en-

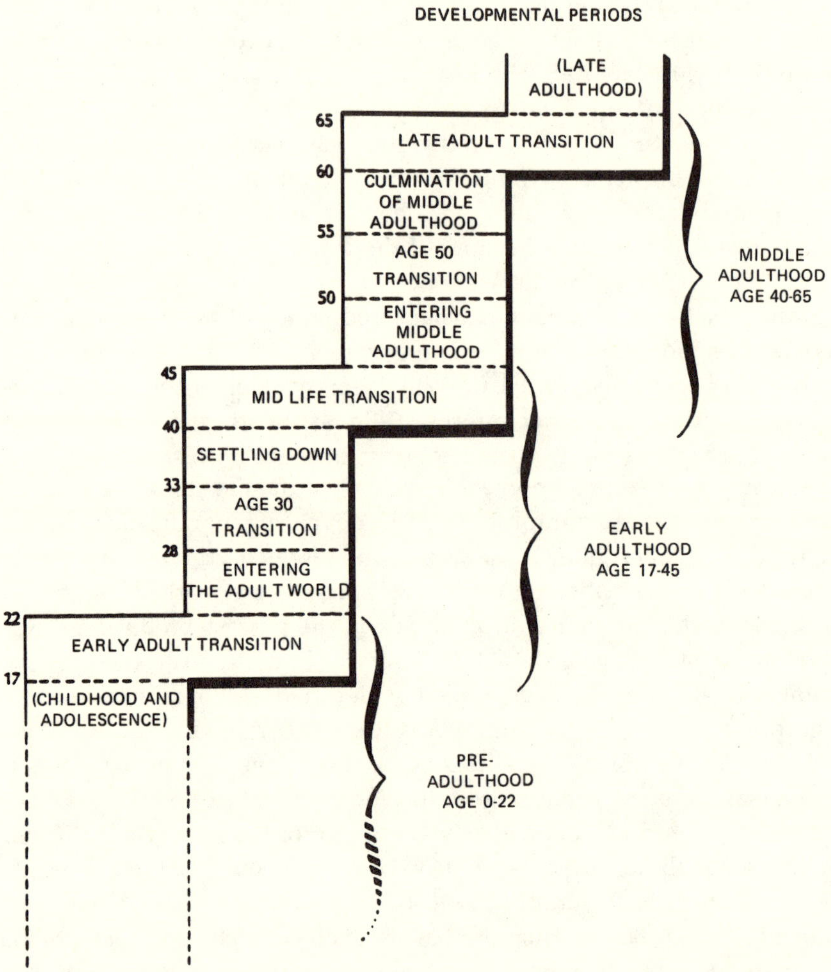

DEVELOPMENTAL PERIODS

FIGURE 2. Eras and developmental periods in early and middle adulthood.

riching his life within it. During intervening transitional periods of four to five years, existing life structures are modified or fundamentally changed in preparation for the next period.

The developmental tasks of the early adult transition (ages 17–22) are to resolve the issues of preadulthood (adolescence) and begin the process of early adulthood by further resolving the dependence of adolescence and trying to establish the self-reliance of early adulthood. Various suitable settings for such tasks exist in society, such as student

TABLE II. *Individual and Marital Stages of Development*[a]

	Stage 1 (18–21 years)	Stage 2 (22–28 years)	Stage 3 (29–31 years)	Stage 4 (32–39 years)	Stage 5 (40–42 years)	Stage 6 (43–59 years)	Stage 7 (60 years and over)
Individual stage	Pulling up roots	Provisional adulthood	Transition at age 30	Settling down	Midlife transition	Middle adulthood	Older age
Individual task	Developing autonomy	Developing intimacy and occupational identification: "getting into the adult world"	Deciding about commitment to work and marriage	Deepening commitments; pursuing more long-range goals	Searching for "fit" between aspirations and environment	Reestablishing and reordering priorities	Dealing effectively with aging, illness, and death while retaining zest for life
Marital task	Shift from family of origin to new commitment	Provisional marital commitment	Commitment crisis: restlessness	Productivity: children, work, friends, and marriage	Summing up: success and failure are evaluated and future goals sought	Resolving conflicts and stabilizing the marriage for the long haul	Supporting and enhancing each other's struggle for productivity and fulfillment in face of the threats of aging
Marital conflict	Original family ties conflict with adaptation	Uncertainty about choice of marital partner: stress over parenthood	Doubts about choice come into sharp conflict: rates of growth may diverge if spouse has not successfully negotiated stage 2 because of parental obligations	Husband and wife have different and conflicting ways of achieving productivity	Husband and wife perceive "success" differently: conflict between individual success and remaining in the marriage	Conflicting rates and directions of emotional growth: concerns about losing youthfulness may lead to depression and/or acting out	Conflicts are generated by rekindled fears of desertion, loneliness, and sexual failure
Intimacy	Fragile intimacy	Deepening but ambivalent intimacy	Increasing distance while partners make up their minds about each other	Marked increase in intimacy in "good" marriages: gradual distancing in "bad" marriages	Tenuous intimacy as fantasies about others increase	Intimacy is threatened by aging and by boredom vis-à-vis a secure and stable relationship: departure of children may increase or decrease intimacy	Struggle to maintain intimacy in the face of eventual separation: in most marriages this dimension achieves a stable plateau
Power	Testing of power	Establishment of patterns of conflict resolution	Sharp vying for power and dominance	Establishment of definite patterns of decision making and dominance	Power in outside world is tested vis-à-vis power in the marriage	Conflicts often increase when children leave, and security appears threatened	Survival fears stir up needs for control and dominance
Marital boundaries	Conflicts over in-laws	Friends and potential lovers: work versus family	Temporary disruptions including extramarital sex or reactive "fortress building"	Nuclear family closes boundaries	Disruption due to reevaluation: drive versus restabilization	Boundaries are usually fixed except in crises such as illness, death, job change, and sudden shift in role relationships	Loss of family and friends leads to closing in of boundaries: physical environment is crucial in maintaining ties with the outside world

[a] From Berman and Lief, 1975.

or apprentice in the university, the business world, the armed forces, and, for some, mental-health training. Levinson points out that many young people, in the midst of this difficult transition, present themselves at clinics, and it is

> crucial that clinicians take the adult development context into account here lest we over-reify the young person's psychopathology and use our expert authority to confirm him in a psychiatric sick role identity. (Newton & Levinson, 1979, p. 489)

The adult world is formally entered when the young man in his twenties (22–28) builds the first adult life structure by choosing an occupation and entering into love relationships, frequently including marriage and family. Two aspects of these developmental tasks are sometimes felt as contrasting or antithetical. On the one hand the individual must *explore* the available possibilities—that is, discover and generate alternative options; and at the same time he must *create a stable structure*—"grow up, get married, enter an occupation, define his goals and lead a more organized life" (Levinson, Darrow, Klein, Levinson, & McKee, 1978, p. 79). So the distinctive character of this developmental period lies in the coexistence of its two tasks: "to explore, to expand one's horizons and put off making firmer commitments until the options are clearer; and to create an initial adult life structure, to have roots, stability, and continuity" (Levinson *et al.*, 1978, p. 80). Most men find a way to balance the need for exploration and stable structure; for example, through stability in work while exploring possibilities in love relationships, or vice versa.

The developmental task of the age-30 transition (ages 28–33) is to question and modify the structure set in place during years 22–28. This is the transition period between entering the adult world in the twenties and settling down in the thirties, "a span of several years in which to reappraise the past and consider the future. He asks: What have I done with my life? What do I want to make of it? What new directions shall I choose?" (Levinson *et al.*, 1978, p. 84). The research showed that all men seem to make some changes during this period, although there is considerable individual variation. For some it is a matter of deepening and extending their initial life structure; for those who find their first life structure flawed, it is a period of considerable developmental crisis and turmoil as change is attempted. Even a person whose life structure has not yet incorporated committed love relationships or occupational focus feels, around the age-30 transition, an acute need to build a more stable, complete life structure.

This occurs during the thirties (33–40), when the early-middle-aged man builds a second life structure for the culmination of early adulthood. This is a time for settling down, for becoming one's own man and achieving youthful dreams and aspirations. At the start of this period a man is on the bottom rung of his career ladder, and during it he moves toward seniority in his line of work or organization. Around age 36 or 37, the approach of success and seniority can provoke a developmental crisis in some since that progress brings not only new rewards, but the burden of increased pressures and responsibilities.

Not infrequently, as part of consolidating their own identities, individuals give up or markedly change their relationships to significant mentors. This is the time when a man joins the tribe as a full adult, finding his niche and assuming greater commitment and responsibility in society, raising a family, and exercising his occupation. This includes community, religio-ethnic group and professional activities.

During the midlife transition, ages 40–45, most men in the study actively questioned the life structures of their thirties, asking such questions as: What have I done with my life? What do I really get from and give to others? What do I truly want for myself? What are my central values and greatest talents? Are they being used or wasted? Have I realized my early Dream?

As in every transitional period, individuation proceeds as the person forms a stronger sense of who he is and what he wants; he forms a clearer boundary between himself and the world. Midlife individuation involves confronting and integrating four pairs of polarities: feelings of youth vs. age, of destructiveness vs. creativity, of masculinity vs. femininity, and of attachment vs. separateness.

> Every life structure necessarily gives high priority to certain aspects of the self and neglects or minimizes other aspects. . . . In the Midlife Transition these neglected parts of the self urgently seek expression. A man experiences them as 'other voices in other rooms' (in Truman Capote's evocative phrase). Internal voices that have been muted for years now clamor to be heard. At times they are heard as a vague whispering, the content unclear but the tone indicating grief over lost opportunities, outrage over betrayal by others, or guilt over betrayal by oneself. At other times they come through as a thunderous roar, the content all too clear, stating names and times and places and demanding that something be done to right the balance. A man hears the voice of an identity prematurely rejected; of a love

> lost or not pursued; of a valued interest or relationship given up in acquies-
> cence to parental or other authority; of an internal figure who wants to be
> an athlete or nomad or artist, to marry for love or remain a bachelor, to get
> rich, enter the clergy or live a sensual carefree life—possibilities set aside
> earlier to become what he now is. *During the midlife transition he must learn to*
> *listen more attentively to these voices and decide consciously what part he will give*
> *them in his life.* (Levinson *et al.*, 1978, p. 200, italics added)

About 80% of the men in the study experienced considerable struggle with self and the external world; their midlife transition was a true developmental crisis. As in the other transitional periods, the clinician who understands the tasks and normative conflicts of this period is better able to help the troubled individual in a reflective and measured way. Labeling men in midlife transition as "irrational," "sick," or "pathologically upset" is neither accurate nor helpful. The desires to question their life structure and possibly change or modify it probably stem from healthy parts of the self. However, this is a critical period in adult development, for the midlife transition can lead either to greater personal individuation with much creative potential or to stagnation and psychological decomposition.

The Yale study concludes with the period from 45–50, when the task is to build an initial structure for middle adulthood. By and large the men in the study had made certain provisional choices in the midlife transition period and now seemed ready to commit themselves to these choices and create new structures during the next seven-year era. The research group believed that the alternation of transitional and stable periods continues for the rest of the life cycle.

GEORGE E. VAILLANT AND *ADAPTATION TO LIFE*

Longitudinal studies of adult development, although most desirable, are undeniably difficult from both methodological and financial standpoints. These difficulties make the Grant Study of Adult Development all the more exceptional. George Vaillant is the current director of the Grant Study, which was begun at Harvard in 1939, and his book *Adaptation to Life* (1977) elaborates what three decades of that study had to teach about how its subjects came of age. The Grant Study was originally conceived because although

> large endowments have been given . . . for the study of the ill, the mentally
> and physically handicapped . . . very few have thought it pertinent to make

a systematic inquiry into the kinds of people who are well and do well. (Heath, 1945, p. 4)

Between 1939 and 1944, 268 male undergraduates were chosen for the study, essentially on the basis of possession of the capacity for self-reliance. These men have now been followed for 40 years, by a series of intermittent interviews supplemented by annual questionnaires. Over 90% have founded stable families, and almost all have achieved occupational distinction. As described by Vaillant, participation in the study has significantly affected the lives of the participants.

Set off by itself in a small brick building, the Study was a warm and friendly place; the staff, from the secretaries to the medical director, were kind and receptive, not analytic and austere. The Grant Study subjects were examined with their full consent and awareness, but they could not volunteer—a condition that helped exclude the quirks of would-be guinea pigs. Because the men were chosen on the grounds of mental health, membership was regarded as a mild honor. Because the staff were interested enough in the men to know when they hurt, the staff were often called upon to give help when it was needed. Thus a strong alliance was forged that has survived for four decades. Most of the men found being part of the Study entertaining and valuable; they acknowledged this freely. A few parents even thought that participation in the project was the most valuable experience that occurred during their son's college career. (p. 41)

For his 1977 volume, Vaillant selected 95 men whom he could interview extensively. Unstructured and free flowing, the interviews were attempts to understand what these men had become; to determine "what had gone right in their lives—not . . . what had gone wrong" (p. 46). The interviews and previous collected material generated many findings and useful conclusions, among them a general confirmation of Erikson's concept of the life cycle. The men who were able to engage the issues of intimacy in their thirties and generativity in their forties had more successful life outcomes than those who were unable to do so. However, an important finding in the study was that despite the achievement of a stable family and occupational success, none of the men had clear sailing; what distinguished effective adaptation was how problems were dealt with, not the absence of problems.

Vaillant's study of adaptation focused on ego mechanisms of defense, the well-known intrapsychic styles of adaptation first described by Freud. Freud recognized most of the defense mechanisms that we understand today and identified their most important properties: Defenses are a major means of managing instinct and affect. They are un-

TABLE III. *Hierarchy of Adaptive Mechanisms*[a]

Level I: Psychotic mechanisms (common in psychosis, dreams, childhood)
  Denial (of external reality)
  Distortion
  Delusional projection
Level II: Immature mechanisms (common in severe depression, personality disorders, and adolescence)
  Fantasy (schizoid withdrawal, denial through fantasy)
  Projection
  Hypochondriasis
  Passive-aggressive behavior (masochism, turning against the self)
  Acting out (compulsive delinquency, perversion)
Level III: Neurotic mechanisms (common in everyone)
  Intellectualization (isolation, obsessive behavior, undoing, rationalization)
  Repression
  Reaction formation
  Displacement (conversion, phobias, wit)
  Dissociation (neurotic denial)
Level IV: Mature mechanisms (common in "healthy" adults)
  Sublimation
  Altruism
  Suppression
  Anticipation
  Humor

---

[a] After Vaillant, 1977, p. 80.

conscious, discrete from one another, dynamic, and reversible and can be adaptive as well as pathological. Building on Freud, Vaillant devised a theoretical hierarchy, grouping 18 defenses according to their *relative maturity* and pathological import (see Table III).

Central to Vaillant's work is the thesis that if individuals are to master conflict gracefully and to harness instinctual strivings creatively, adaptive styles, that is, ego mechanisms of defense, *must mature throughout the life cycle.* In the Grant-Study subjects, with the passage of years, *mature defenses were used with relatively greater frequency.* As adolescents the Grant-Study men were twice as likely to use immature defenses as mature ones; as young adults they were twice as likely to use mature mechanisms as immature ones. In midlife they were four times as likely to use mature as immature defenses.

In looking at the change in specific defenses over time, the Vaillant research group traced the decline of the defense mechanisms of fantasy

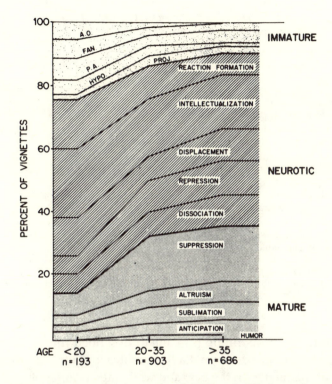

FIGURE 3. Shifts in defensive styles during the adult life cycle. The figure shows the distribution of defensive vignettes shown by 95% of subjects at adolescence, young adulthood, and middle age. AO indicates acting out; FAN, fantasy; PA, passive aggression; HYPO, hypochondriasis, PROJ, projection. Reprinted from Vaillant, 1977, p. 331 by permission.

and acting out with maturity and a concomitant increase in suppression. Dissociation, repression, sublimation, and altruism increase in midlife, while projection, hypochondriasis, and masochism are most common in adolescence. Vaillant also points out that the decade from 25 to 35 is a guilty period in which defenses of reaction formation and repression are used with greater frequency (Figure 3).

Vaillant compared men who were considered generative, that is, more psychosocially mature in Eriksonian terms, with a group of "perpetual boys." Over time the perpetual boys failed to show any significant shift in their adaptive patterns, quite unlike the pattern seen in the generative men.

TABLE IV. *Differences between Best and Worst Outcomes Relevant to an Eriksonian Model of the Life Cycle*[a]

	Best outcomes (30 men)	Worst outcomes (30 men)
Childhood environment poor	17%	47%[b]
Pessimism, self-doubt, passivity, and fear of sex at 50	3%	50%[c]
In college personality integration put in bottom fifth	0	33%[b]
Subjects whose career choice reflected identification with father	60%	27%[b]
Dominated by mother in adult life	0	40%[c]
Failure to marry by 30	3%	37%[b]
Bleak friendship patterns by 50	0	57%[c]
Current job has little supervisory responsibility	20%	93%[c]
Children admitted to father's college	47%	10%[b]
Children's outcome described as good or excellent	66%	23%[b]
Average yearly charitable contribution	$3,000	$500

[a] From Vaillant, 1977, p. 350.
[b] Significant difference ($p < .03$—a difference that would occur by chance only 1 time in 33).
[c] Very significant difference ($p < .001$—a difference that would occur by chance only 1 time in 1000).

Summing up his findings, Vaillant described the association between maturation and external adjustment. He contrasted the relative success of the men with the best and worst life outcomes in negotiating the stages of the Eriksonian life cycle. Those with best outcomes were able to negotiate the various stages of the life cycle with considerable more success than those with worst outcomes (Table IV). Difficulties for those with worst outcomes started in childhood; blind raters described their early childhoods as traumatic, interfering with the establishment of basic trust, autonomy, and initiative. Vaillant suggests that

> their mistrust of themselves and of their universe persisted into adult life;
> for behavior vignettes reflecting pessimism, self-doubt, and fear of sex were
> far more frequent in the adult lives of the Worst Outcomes. (pp. 349–350)

These men were seen as less integrated in adolescence, and subsequently their identities were less secure as adults. Interestingly, they were also less likely to have internalized their fathers as role models and still seemed quite dependent on their mothers. Finally, both at 30 and 50 they were still having trouble with intimacy. Their marriages and friendships were problematic, and they seemed to be considerably less generative in the sense of being willing to assume responsibility for other adults.

The Grant Study demonstrates the tremendous value of longitudinal study in the field of adult development, pointing out not only that individuals grow during their entire lives but also *how* they grow. The change in ego defense patterns from adolescence to midlife is convincing evidence that intrapsychic structural change occurs throughout the adult years.

Roger L. Gould and *Transformations*

Roger Gould was one of the first psychiatrists to recognize a predictable sequence of changing patterns and preoccupations during the adult years. In an early study, he and his colleagues observed and studied group-psychotherapy patients in the UCLA outpatient department. After discounting problems common to all age groups (e.g., anxiety and depression), patterns specific to the age groups emerged. This study then led to a project, reported in the *American Journal of Psychiatry* in 1972, called "The Phases of Adult Life: A Study in Developmental Psychology." Using a questionnaire incorporating salient statements about the age-related feelings of the treatment group, Gould and his research group asked 524 nonpatients from 16 to 50 to rank the statements in relation to themselves. Patients and nonpatients of the same age had roughly the *same* general concerns about living, which were quite specific for their age.

In his book *Transformations: Growth and Change in Adult Life* (1978), Gould outlined the developmental steps in which adult consciousness is gradually achieved by understanding and overcoming the childhood consciousness that invades our adult lives and interferes with developmental progression. An aspect of that infantile remnant involves "demonic anger," an overestimation of the power of hostility in ourselves and others.

> By striving for a fuller, more independent adult consciousness, we trigger the angry demons of childhood consciousness. Growing and reformulating our self-definition becomes a dangerous act. It is the act of transformation. (p. 25)

So adult consciousness progresses by mastering childhood fear as the adult learns to understand and modulate the childhood anger released by change in the course of confronting the new developmental tasks of adulthood. Underlying every new self-defining issue in adult life is an unconscious, restrictive set of "protective devices" which form a boundary of safety. Thus in the process of self-definition we must traverse a "moat of terror" and abandon the childhood illusion of absolute safety.

The protective devices, which themselves change and evolve (as do the ego mechanisms of defense which Vaillant described), include irrational acts, rigid childhood rules, fantasy, and a number of *false assumptions*. All support the four basic assumptions of childhood which are contained in the illusion of absolute safety:

1. We'll always live with our parents and be their child.
2. They'll always be there to help when we can't do something on our own.
3. Their simplified version of our complicated inner reality is correct, as when they turn the light on in our bedroom to prove there are no ghosts.
4. There is no real death or evil in the world. (p. 39)

By the time one enters young adulthood (at the end of high school), these assumptions are abandoned intellectually, but unconsciously they continue to play an important part in adult experience. The gradual shedding of these immature beliefs makes possible the shift from childhood to adult consciousness and is at the center of Gould's thinking about adult development.

He divides adult experience into four chronological eras, similar to the divisions made by Erikson and Levinson. Each era has its own major false assumption and a number of false subassumptions—its own developmental tasks and conflicts—which must be challenged and mastered.

LEAVING OUR PARENTS' WORLD, ages 16–22
Major false assumption: "I'll always belong to my parents and believe in their world." (pp. 47–48)
Component false assumptions:
1. If I get any more independent, it will be a disaster.
2. I can see the world only through my parents' assumptions.
3. Only my parents can guarantee my safety.
4. My parents must be my only family.
5. I don't own my own body. (p. 48)

I'M NOBODY'S BABY NOW, ages 22–28:
Major false assumption: "Doing things my parents' way, with will-power and perseverance, will bring results. But if I become too frustrated,

confused or tired or am simply unable to cope, they will step in and show me the right way." (pp. 75–76)

Component false assumptions:

1. Rewards will come automatically if we do what we are supposed to do.
2. There is only one right way to do things.
3. Those in a special relationship with us can do for us what we haven't been able to do for ourself.
4. Rationality, commitment, and effort will always prevail over all other forces. (p. 76)

OPENING UP TO WHAT'S INSIDE—ages 28–34:

Major false assumption: "Life is simple and controllable. There are no significant coexisting contradictory forces within me." (p. 153)

Component false assumptions:

1. What I know intellectually, I know emotionally.
2. I am not like my parents in ways I don't want to be.
3. I can see the reality of those close to me quite clearly.
4. Threats to my security aren't real. (p. 164)

MIDLIFE DECADE—ages 35–45:

Major false assumption: "There is no evil or death in the world. The sinister has been destroyed." (p. 217)

Component false assumptions:

1. The illusion of safety can last forever.
2. Death can't happen to me or my loved ones.
3. It's impossible to live without a protector (women).
4. There is no life beyond this family.
5. I am an innocent. (p. 219)

Gould concludes that adult consciousness becomes realized to the extent that we challenge and master these false assumptions from childhood consciousness. However, if we tie ourselves too closely to our protective illusions and try to remain absolutely safe we do not take the risks necessary to emancipate ourselves from childhood consciousness, and the danger of stagnation exists.

Bernice L. Neugarten and the Chicago School of Human Development

For over a decade, Bernice Neugarten and her colleagues of the Committee on Human Development at the University of Chicago (Neugarten, 1975) have carried out numerous studies in the field of personality development in middle and later life; research on adaptational patterns, career lines, age norms, and age-appropriate behaviors in adults, and on attitudes and values across generational lines. Some 2,000 normal adults have participated in these related investigations in samples of 100 to 200, usually drawn from the metropolitan communities of Chicago and Kansas City.

Neugarten, an avid spokesperson for a psychology of adulthood, has metaphorically described efforts to study the adult. Together under the circus big top, child psychologists sit too close to the entrance while gerontologists congregate near the exit. Thus "both groups are missing a view of the whole show," leaving us without sufficient understanding of the adult (Neugarten, 1975, p. 378). The data available on individuals who have been studied from childhood into adulthood are disproportionately weighted to the early years, emphasizing the variables most salient in childhood, and inadequate to yield theories that would have central relevance for adult behavior. She states the case well:

> Where, except perhaps to certain ego psychologists who use terms such as "competence," "self," and "effectance," can we look for concepts to describe the incredible complexity shown in the behavior of a business executive, age fifty, who makes a thousand decisions in the course of a day? What terms shall we use to describe the strategies with which such a person manages his time, buffers himself from certain stimuli, makes elaborate plans and schedules, sheds some of his "load" by delegating some tasks to other people over whom he has certain forms of control, accepts other tasks as being singularly appropriate to his own competencies and responsibilities, and in the same twenty-four-hour period, succeeds in satisfying his emotional and sexual and aesthetic needs?
>
> It is the incongruity between existing psychological concepts and theories, on the one hand, and the transactions that constitute everyday adult behavior, on the other, to which I am drawing attention. (p. 384)

The Salient Issues in Adulthood

From lengthy interviews with 100 men and women aged 45 to 55, selected on the basis of success in their careers or visibility in civic affairs, the following issues emerged as typical of middle adulthood, appearing in different forms, if at all, in younger or older people.

(a) Middle-aged adults look to themselves as the instrument through which to achieve a form of "self-utilization."

(b) Because of an increased sense of physical vulnerability, protective strategies are devised to maintain the body—a form of "body monitoring."

(c) Increasingly, time is viewed in terms of time-left-to-live rather than time-since-birth.

(d) Death becomes personalized, applying to loved ones and particularly to oneself.

(e) A new perspective and increased self-understanding comes from being a part of the middle generation, in a position to observe both the younger and older generations objectively.

(f) Because of realized expertise, ongoing accomplishment is felt to be appropriate and expected.

(g) Taking stock, reflecting, structuring and restructuring experience, indeed, all aspects of introspection take on increased importance.

Changes in Personality in the Second Half of Life

Although not longitudinal, these studies have delineated processes of change characteristic of middle age (Neugarten *et al.*, 1964). The Chicago group introduces an important concept in adult development which they call "increased interiority of the personality" (Neugarten *et al.*, 1964). Beginning in midlife with a tendency toward increased self-reflection and introspection (most heightened in the decade of the fifties), the phenomenon becomes even more marked in later life, leading to what Butler (1963) calls the "life review," the increased reminiscence of the aged, which Butler believes is a universal occurrence and may lead to dramatic changes in the personalities of older people. Related to interiority of the personality is a decrease in "ego energy" and a shift in "ego style." The older person tends to respond to inner rather than outer stimuli, to withdraw emotional investments, to give up some measure of self-assertiveness, and to utilize a passive, magical style of ego functioning.

There is some evidence for a change in sex-role perception in the second half of life. Older men (55–70), in contrast to younger men (40–54), tend to feel more submissive toward women, whereas older women evolve in a more authoritative direction, reversing roles in the family. An additional finding confirms Jung's observation (see Chapter 2) that women as they age become more comfortable with their aggressive and assertive impulses, while men develop greater acceptance of their nurturing and affiliative impulses. However, in both sexes older people move toward more egocentric, self-preoccupied positions and attend increasingly to the control and satisfaction of personal needs (Neugarten, 1975, p. 385).

Neugarten and her group have made a very significant contribution to the study of adult development through persistent and long-standing efforts to collect behavioral data from rather large groups of people, calling attention to the network of age norms and expectations that govern behavior and affect the relationships among age groups. These norms and expectations are part of an elaborate, pervasive social attitude toward middle and old age which greatly influences the course of adult development during these phases of life.

ROBERT J. LIFTON: DEATH AWARENESS AND THE IMAGE OF CONTINUITY

Robert Lifton, a psychiatrist and psychohistorian, in a series of remarkable books and studies (*History and Human Survival*, 1970; *Home from the War*, 1973; *Death in Life*, 1976a; *The Life of the Self*, 1976b; and *The Broken Connection*, 1979), has brought attention to the contemporary awareness of death and the human need for a sense of continuity. In Lifton's opinion, Americans have awakened to the importance of death and anxiety about death, but "more elusive has been the psychological relationship between the phenomenon of death and the flow of life" (1979, p. 4). His studies have focused on humans in extreme situations: victims of the Holocaust, Hiroshima, Vietnam. As a result of his work he has perceived a historical shift in our anxieties "from Victorian struggles concerning sexuality and moralism to our present preoccupation with absurd death (and by implication, absurd life) and unlimited technological violence" (1979, p. 4).

> The broken connection exists in the tissues of our mental life. It has to do with a very new historical—one could also say evolutionary—relationship to death. We are haunted by the image of exterminating ourselves as a species by means of our own technology. (1979, p. 5)

Central to Lifton's discussion are three aspects of knowledge related to man's evolution: He knows that he will die; he has the capacity to symbolize; he is able to create culture. Lifton disagrees with Freud and Rank, who believed that culture arises from the need to deny death. He thinks of human culture rather as a

> way of living out this unique awareness that [man] both dies and continues
> . . . "knowledge," in our sense, is the capacity of the symbolizing imagina-
> tion to explore the idea of death and relate it to a principle of life—
> continuity—that is, the capacity for culture. (1979, p. 7)

Lifton has applied his ideas to the life cycle and specifically to adulthood. Integration, or a balance of immediate fulfillment and ultimate connectedness, grows from the adult's capacity to be aware of death without being incapacitated by anxiety about it. The image of death, what Erikson calls "an ego chill," a shudder attending the awareness of our possible nonexistence, is for the most part suppressed in American culture during young adulthood. However, Lifton and many other researchers, including ourselves, find that sometime during the late thirties and early forties thoughts of one's own death persistently intrude into consciousness. Tasks are carried out in a struggle against time, with a sense of "now or never." Death imagery is particularly relevant to midlife crisis.

> The process can take the form of a low-key self-questioning, or it can be
> filled with pain and suffering. But it now seems that some period of conflict
> is a regular aspect of the adult phase of the life cycle, at least in our society.
> One can speak of an endless wave of death imagery that, building in inten-
> sity, causes endless anxiety. Having been so long suppressed, this imagery
> can break out and overwhelm consciousness. (Lifton, 1979, p. 88)

Yet total suppression of such feelings brings risks of stagnation, accompanied by what Lifton calls a "numbing feeling." In contradistinction, men and women are able to allow the anxieties to come to the surface, and to deal with them creatively. Lifton complains that psychological theory has neglected the seasoning and experience which an individual in his forties can bring to a creative consolidation and resolution of these midlife experiences:

> There is a special quality of life-power available only to those seasoned
> by struggles of four or more decades. That seasoning includes extensive cul-
> tivation of images and forms having to do with love and caring, with expe-
> rienced parenthood, with teaching and mentorship, with work combina-
> tions and professional creativity, with responses to intellectual and artistic
> images around one, and above all with humor and a sense of the absurd.
> The seasoned psychic forms are by no means devoid of death imagery.
> Rather they are characterized by ingenious combinations of death equiva-
> lents and immediate affirmations, or melancholic recognition of the
> fragmentation and threat surrounding all ultimate involvements, along with
> dogged insistence upon one's own connections beyond the self—one's own
> relationship to collective modes of symbolic immortality. Like the despair,
> the life-power of this stage can be especially profound. (1979, pp. 88–89)

GEORGE H. POLLOCK: THE MOURNING PROCESS AND CREATIVITY

Among contemporary developmental psychoanalysts, George Pollock's approach is most similar to our own. For 20 years he has studied different facets of the mourning process and has found that the process serves as an adaptation to various losses throughout life. Bereavement is only one instance of mourning, a process which can follow not only death, but loss, disappointment, or change, and is a normal part of lifelong development. Having observed mourning and its relationship to anniversary phenomena, time, trauma, affects, utopian quests, and the creative process, and documented it in all cultures, in all the religions, and throughout time, Pollock (1979) asserts that

> mourning is a universal transformational process that allows us to accept a reality that exists, which may be different from our wishes and hopes, which recognizes loss and change, both externally and internally, and which . . . can result in a happier life, fulfilled and fulfilling for ourselves and for others. For the gifted the mourning process may be part of or the end-product that can result in creativity in art, music, literature, science, philosophy, religion. (ms. p. 10)

Thus Pollock describes a mechanism for development; that is, change in adulthood is facilitated by the transformational, adaptive process of mourning, and the outcome may be creative.

Pollock does not share Freud's pessimism about analyzing older individuals, and he has begun to describe treatment experiences and strategies for people in the second half of life. Freud (1932) stated that one factor that impaired the therapeutic effectiveness of psychoanalysis with older people was the amount of psychical rigidity; as people get older there is " . . . a general stiffening of mental life; the psychical processes, to which one could very well indicate other paths, seem incapable of abandoning the older ones" (p. 154). Fenichel (1945) went further, suggesting that the optimal age range for psychoanalysis was from 15 to 40, and that after 40 psychoanalytic treatment may be counterindicated. This has not been Dr. Pollock's experience, or, as he points out, that of a number of other analysts. Pearl King noted that narcissistic threats to middle-aged and aged patients, including the physical, psychological, and social effects of aging, bring a sense of urgency and motivation to their treatment that helps establish a productive therapeutic alliance. In her experience, when therapy is successful older patients may begin to find new forms of creativity within themselves and unexpected satisfactions.

In his own experiences, Pollock finds a particular therapeutic benefit from free association, dream reporting, and fantasizing in the elderly because they

> feel in control and have some competence in being able to do what is requested, they achieve relief from the cathartic expression of feelings and concern, there is diminished sense of isolation and loneliness, and when they can establish linkages between inside and outside and past and present there is therapeutic progress that stimulates the process even further. (1979, ms. pp. 52–53)

Pollock's work with older patients has provided an important contribution to the theory of treatment technique: the reversal of transference feelings. At times an elderly patient may relate to the analyst as if he or she were the son or daughter who "understands, is interested, is trustworthy, is protective and supportive" (p. 53). Although there may be some actual fulfilling of a son's protective role with an elderly patient, for the most part Pollock uses his usual interpretive approach and such patients are able to relieve their tension and anxiety through analytic understanding. Likewise, in working with the aged the therapist's countertransference attitudes and feelings are significant. Older patients are often quick to detect the therapist's mood.

He has found, especially in dealing with older patients, that the focus on the mourning process is important:

> The basic loss is the loss of parts of the self that once were, that one hoped might be but will not any longer and with the working out of these mournings for lost self, others, hopes, aspirations, and other losses and changes, there is an ability to face reality as it is and as it can be changed to provide a greater quality of life. Newer sublimations, interests, activities can appear. There can be new relationships with old objects as well as with new objects. Past truly can become past and distinguished from present and future. (1979, ms. p. 54)

Thus many different aspects of learning are possible for elderly patients in psychotherapy and psychoanalysis. Insight, educational improvement from support and relationship, and identification with the therapist all occur. The reappearance of sexual feelings in reality, dreams, and in fantasies has positive implications for an "investment in life." In some instances the reestablishment of sexual relations is not only a return to the past, but indicates creative freedom in the present. Pollock asserts (and we agree) that "the capacity for developing a transference neurosis is present regardless of the age of the individual [and] catharsis, confrontation, insight, and interpretation are useful" in psychotherapeutic work with people of all ages (1979, p. 58). In view of the increased numbers of people in the second half of life, it is gratifying to realize that the psychotherapeutic methods we have on hand, or an elaboration of those methods, promise considerable benefit.

REFERENCES

Berman, E. M., & Lief, H. I. Marital therapy from a psychiatric perspective: An overview. *American Journal of Psychiatry*, 1975, *132*, 6.

Butler, R. N. The life review: An interpretation of reminiscence in the aged. *Psychiatry*, 1963, *26*, 65.

Fenischel, O. *The psychoanalytic theory of neurosis*. New York: W. W. Norton, 1945.

Freud, S. *New introductory lectures on psycho-analysis*. Standard edition 22:3. London: Hogarth Press, 1932.

Gould, R. L. The phases of adult life: A study in developmental psychology. *American Journal of Psychiatry*, 1972, *129*, 521.

Gould, R. L. *Transformations: Growth and change in adult life*. New York: Simon & Schuster, 1978.

Heath, C. W. *What people are*. Cambridge: Harvard University Press, 1945.

Levinson, D. J., Darrow, C. N., Klein, E. B., Levinson, M. H., & McKee, B. *The seasons of a man's life*. New York: Alfred A. Knopf, 1978.

Lifton, R. J. Protean man (pp. 311–331). The young and the old: Notes on a new history (pp. 332–373). *History and human survival*. New York: Random House, 1970.

Lifton, R. J. *Home from the war*. New York: Simon & Schuster, 1973.

Lifton, R. J. *Death in life*. New York: Touchstone Books, 1976. (a)

Lifton, R. J. *The life of the self*. New York: Simon & Schuster, 1976. (b)

Lifton, R. J. *The broken connection*. New York: Simon & Schuster, 1979.

Neugarten, B. L. Adult personality: Toward a psychology of the life cycle. In W. C. Sze (Ed.), *The human life cycle*. New York: Jason Aronson, 1975.

Neugarten, B. L. Time, age, and the life cycle. *American Journal of Psychiatry*, 1979, *136*, 887.

Neugarten, B. L., with Berkowitz, H., Crotty, W. J., Gruen, W., Gutmann, D. L., Lubin, M. I., Miller, D. L., Peck, R. F., Rosen, J. L., Shukin, A., & Tobin, S. S. *Personality in middle and late life*. New York: Atherton Press, 1964.

Newton, P. M., & Levinson, D. J. Crisis in adult development. In A. Lazare (Ed.), *Outpatient psychiatry, diagnosis and treatment*. Baltimore: Williams & Wilkins, 1979.

Pollock, G. H. *Aging or aged: Development or pathology?* Unpublished manuscript, 1979.

Stevens-Long, J. *Adult life: Developmental processes*. Palo Alto, Calif.: Mayfield, 1979.

Vaillant, G. E. *Adaptation to life*. Boston: Little, Brown, 1977.

II
NEW CONCEPTS

4

Hypotheses about the Psychodynamic Theory of Adult Development

When I was younger, there was much talk about the century of the child. Has it ended? We hope it has quietly joined the era. Since then we have gone through something like a century of youth. But when, pray, is the century of the adult to begin?

Eric Erikson, 1974

Psychoanalysis has not formulated a comprehensive theory of normal adult development. Sophisticated and detailed with regard to childhood and adolescence, the theory is sparse for the remainder of the life cycle, in part because the developmental framework has not been applied fully to the study of the adult. Usually adulthood is characterized as a lengthy, stable phase of life in which developmental processes play a relatively minor role.

There is a small body of developmental literature on adulthood, but it has not been elaborated into an organized whole. Among the most significant recent literature is the work of Gould (1978), Levinson, Darrow, Klein, Levinson, and McKee (1978), and Vaillant (1977). In this chapter we will integrate existing theory with clinical data from our own experience and concepts from related fields, forming a set of psychodynamic hypotheses about the nature of the developmental process in the adult.

The basis for this chapter is an article entitled "Some Observations and Hypotheses about the Psychoanalytic Theory of Adult Development," written by the authors and published in the *International Journal of Psycho-Analysis*, 1979, *60*, Part I, 59–71.

59

HISTORY

With the publication of *The Interpretation of Dreams* (1900), *Three Essays on the Theory of Sexuality* (1905), *The Case of Little Hans* (1909) and other works, Freud laid a foundation for psychoanalytic developmental thought. His efforts were directed primarily toward psychopathology, and his hypotheses were based on the idea that intrapsychic conflict was the major stimulus to psychic growth; an idea which persisted until the appearance of *Ego Psychology and the Problem of Adaptation* (Hartmann, 1939/1958). The addition of Hartmann's concept of primary autonomy—the emergence of certain mental functions outside the sphere of conflict—added a new dimension to the understanding of development and moved psychoanalysis toward a general psychology of human behavior, a goal only partially realized in regard to adult behavior. Hartmann said:

> We must recognize that though the ego certainly does grow on conflicts, these are not the only roots of ego development. Many of us expect psychoanalysis to become a general *developmental psychology*; to do so, it must encompass these other roots of ego development . . . . This naturally gives new importance to the direct observation of developmental processes by psychoanalysts. (p. 8)

Thus in the 1930s and 1940s, on the basis of understanding provided by Freud, the emergence of ego psychology, and the maturation of child psychoanalysis as a discipline, the developmental framework grew to be a significant conceptual tool, and although its application to adulthood has been limited, several significant articles in the literature of the last 30 years give impetus to our current thought.

The contributions of Therese Benedek (1950) deserve special attention in both a historical and a theoretic sense. In an early article she conceptualized parenthood as a developmental phase, emphasizing the roles of such experiences as motherhood and the climacteric as vehicles for growth. By integrating genetic and organic factors with current experience she presented a balanced view of the dynamic forces that determine psychic development in the adult. Take, for example, this quotation:

> Motherhood, indeed, plays a significant role in the development of woman. Physiologically it completes maturation; psychologically, it channelizes the primarily introverted, narcissistic tendencies into many psychic

qualities designated "feminine," such as responsiveness, empathy, sympathy and the desire to do, to care for others, etc. Thus, from motherliness it is only one step to many forms of feminine achievement since these, or many of them, represent the extension and expansion of motherliness. (p. 20)

An article by Leo Rangell (1953) is entitled "The Role of the Parent in the Oedipal Complex" is of historical importance, because in it Rangell explains adult experience in developmental terms, describing the effect of oedipal themes on various aspects of parenthood from the birth of the first child to reactions to a new son- or daughter-in-law. The oedipal complex is seen as a dynamic process evolving with the individual and affecting development throughout the life cycle.

Erikson (1963) was one of the first analysts to attempt a formulation of a developmental theory for the entire life cycle. His ideas are well-known and have had a profound influence on thinking about adulthood. We view his concepts as nodal ideas that have served to stimulate the thinking of those interested in the dynamic development of the adult.

Recently the developmental focus has received increased attention at the meetings of the American Psychoanalytic Association—in particular, from members of panels on "Separation–Individuation throughout the Life Cycle" (Marcus, 1973; Steinschein, 1973; Winestine, 1973); "Parenthood as a Developmental Phase" (Parens, 1975); and the Conference on Psychoanalytic Education and Research, Commission IX report on "Child Analysis" (1974).

Some Hypotheses about Adult Development

We sense now a particular readiness to focus on adult development, and we have formulated seven hypotheses in an initial effort to lay the groundwork for a more comprehensive theory.

Hypothesis I. The Nature of the Development Process Is Basically the Same in the Adult as in the Child

Spitz (1965) defined development as "the emergence of forms, of function and of behaviour which are the outcome of exchanges between the organism on the one hand, the inner and outer environment on the other" (p. 5). Hartmann's (1939/1958) concept of adaptation, which he describes as "primarily a reciprocal relationship between the organism and its environment" (p. 24), holds the same idea. The critical concept contained in both these definitions is that development is the result of the *interaction* between biological organism and environment. One or the other pole may exert more influence, but never to the exclusion of the other.

A commonly held conception is that the adult, compared to the child, is relatively free of environmental influences. Hartmann, for example, speaks of the process of progressive internalization. Internalization may be defined as, "in its broadest aspect, a progressive process by which external interactions between the organism and the outer world are replaced by inner representations of these interactions and their end results" (Moore & Fine, 1968, p. 57). As the organism achieves increased independence from its environment, reactions that originally occurred in relation to the external world are increasingly internalized. Examples of this would be the mastery of bowel and bladder function and the control of motor and mental activities such as riding a bicycle, tying shoes, or reading and writing. This idea is clear in regard to mental and physical activity in childhood, but it does seem to imply that as the human organism moves into adulthood the individual is less dependent on the environment; a notion stated precisely by Eissler (1975):

> In early life periods, biology and the primary demands of reality furnish the guidelines of a necessary development. The guidelines of latency, puberty and adolescence are increasingly defined by demands of culture and sexual maturation. The adult, though, should be more or less free, even though limited by the general biological framework. In the ideal case internal processes are autonomous and are not primarily determined by immediate biological or sociocultural factors, as occurs in the preceding phases of development. (p. 139)

In contradistinction, we suggest that *in the achievement of new and phase-specific developmental tasks of adulthood, the individual is as dependent as the child on the environment.* But in adulthood the environment necessary to promote continued growth changes. For instance, parents are replaced by spouse and children and the play environment is supplemented by, for the most part, the work environment. Normal adult functioning postulates mature sexual activity and the capacity for intimacy, which are impossible without a loved and loving partner. Further, generativity (Erikson's concept of caring for the next generation), although it draws heavily on inner resources, is meaningless without an environment that provides children and young adults to guide and inspire. Creativity and work, even of the most introspective kind as in music, art, and literature are empty unless they interpret human experience in relation to the environment and with others in mind.

To be sure, the degree of psychopathology or health that the individual brings to adulthood influences both the environment he chooses to live in and his response to it; but in either event the continued evolution of mental activity and functioning are strongly influenced by that environment.

> A woman of 32, limited by her neurosis, was unable to form a loving relationship with a man and was living at home with her parents. Through treatment she was able to change her inner environment, the neurosis, and later the outer environment by becoming a wife and mother in addition to having a successful career. If she had remained at home with her parents the environmental prerequisites for confronting, mastering, and integrating developmental tasks such as sexuality, intimacy, and parenthood would have been not present or present in attenuated form. In such a situation she might have continued to grow in certain ways, such as the sublimation of maternal and generative concerns through caring for her aging parents or through her work, but she would not have engaged in those relationships which encourage the broadest forms of development.

Thus, the essence of our point is that exchanges between organism and environment occur from birth to death, producing a continuous effect on psychic development. The adult is not a finished product insulated from the environment but, like the child, is in a state of dynamic tension which continually affects and changes him. From that hypothesis a second follows.

Hypothesis II. Development in Adulthood Is an Ongoing, Dynamic Process

The most prevalent psychoanalytic conception does not hold that adults undergo dynamic development. Anna Freud, Humberto Nagera, and W. Ernest Freud (1965), in their work on the adult profile, wrote:

> In this instance assessment is concerned not with an ongoing process but with a finished product in which, by implication, the ultimate developmental stages should have been reached. The developmental point of view may be upheld only insofar as success or failure to reach this level or to maintain it determines the so-called maturity or immaturity of the adult personality. (p. 10)

This reference from the most distinguished developmental theoreticians using such phrases as "not with an ongoing process but with a finished product," and "the ultimate developmental stages should have been reached" supports the conception of the adult as a static, finished product instead of a dynamic, constantly changing and developing organism.

Psychoanalysis has long recognized the importance of adult experiences such as pregnancy, marriage, aging, death, and so on as issues and crises in their own right, but usually in relationship to past experiences and conflicts. What has not been emphasized enough, we feel, is an emphasis on these experiences as developmental issues in and of themselves, regardless of the past.

Such a developmental viewpoint of adulthood has been presented in a recent article by Morton Shane (1977).

> The developmental *orientation* must be distinguished from the genetic (sometimes called "developmental" or "genetic developmental") *point of view*. Not only is the concept on a lower level of abstraction, closer to the clinical data, but it is also different in that "developmental" implies an ongoing process, not only with a past, but also with a present and a future, while "genetic" is limited to the past, especially in terms of how the past is retrospectively perceived, related to and understood in the present, and is exclusively derived from the analytic situation. The use of the developmental approach implies that the analytic patient, regardless of age, is considered to be still in the process of ongoing development as opposed to merely being in possession of a past that influences his present conscious and unconscious life. (pp. 95–96)

At present these two divergent views of the adult exist side by side in analytic theory. Agreeing with Shane, we see the adult, as we do the child, as in a constant state of dynamic flux and feel that this process is part of the human condition at all ages.

The conceptual bridge between the two viewpoints may be an increased understanding of the *difference* between the developmental processes in the child and the adult, not the *absence* of the developmental process in the adult. One aspect of that difference is reflected in our next hypothesis.

Hypothesis III. Whereas Childhood Development Is Focused Primarily on the Formation of Psychic Structure, Adult Development Is Concerned with the Continuing Evolution of Existing Psychic Structure and with Its Use

Part of the reason the adult has been conceptualized as static may be a failure to recognize the scope and the subtleness of psychic change in adulthood. Whereas the formation of psychic structure in a child is like broad strokes painted on a bare canvas, the evolution of psychic structure in adulthood is equivalent to fine, nearly invisible strokes on a complicated background—a van Gogh compared to a Raphael. The appearance of new and basic mental functions in childhood is easier to notice than the internal refinements in these structures which occur in adulthood.

A specific example of this difference is well illustrated by Binstock in a recent article (1973) in which he compares adolescent infatuation and mature adult love.

> The state of being in love completes the lover's identity as part of a male-female duality. It is a structure-forming state in the ego which aspires to genitality. Whereas infatuation is an exercise in identity formation along the lines of sexual differentiation and sorting out issues about activity and passivity, the gratifying love relationship, by contrast, puts into practice the structuring that has already occurred. *Whereas infatuation ends with being in love, genital love begins with it.* Of course, neither of these generalizations applies in pure form. If the infatuated lover obtains no gratification, his pursuit is a dreary and depressing one. If the adult lover undergoes no further development in the gratifying relationship, the life gradually goes out of it. Love involves a continuing securing and refinement of identity, else it will not endure. (p. 104, italics added)

So adolescent infatuation builds structure and adult love refines it by stimulating a continuous evolution in identity and other processes. Adult love is thus an expression of existing structure and a modifier of it.

Settlage uses the word "rearrangements" (Winestine, 1973, p. 141) to describe this evolution in adulthood, relating it to (a) biologically determined progression through the developmental stages, (b) the gradual shift from the family of origin to the family of procreation (a process that continues well into adult years), and (c) changing technological and sociocultural conditions. Benedek (1975), in describing the same processes, uses the term "psychological reorganization" (p. 338).

To elaborate, let us consider the functioning and evolution of certain mental functions in adulthood. What normally happens to the defense mechanisms, to identifications, and so on as a result of the physical, psychological, and social changes of midlife? What is the developmental line in adulthood of the essentially autonomous ego functions postulated by Hartmann (1939/1958)—that is, perception, intention, thinking, language, recall phenomena, productivity, and motor development? Do they continue to evolve or does their development cease?

As an example of this continued evolution, consider the process of identification. By identification we mean

> an automatic, unconscious mental process whereby an individual becomes like another person in one or several aspects. It is a natural accompaniment of maturation and mental development and aids in the learning process (including the learning of speech and language), as well as in the acquisition of interests, ideals, mannerisms, etc. (Moore & Fine, 1978, p. 50)

In childhood, identification serves multiple functions which promote normal development, such as a little girl assuming her mother's mannerisms or a latency-age boy become an avid baseball fan like his father. We believe that identification continues to further the developmental process in adulthood as well, as exemplified by the mentor relationship.

For many creative scientists a close relationship with an older mentor during their formative, young-adult years is crucial. This new adult identification is central to the scientific commitment and work process which eventually leads to new discoveries. Although in part based on the earlier infantile identifications, such adult processes should not be seen as mere replications of parent–child relationships. The identification with the original objects deals with *how* the child builds psychic structure and becomes like the adult, whereas later identifications provide *specificity* to the adult personality, in this example to the choice of profession and quality of work achievement. The capacity for creativity, the legacy of childhood, is directed into specific areas by the adult identification.

In acquiring an identity as a mental-health professional, students identify with their mentors—teachers, supervisors, and therapists. The identifications are particularly apparent in regard to minute expressions of therapeutic style—frequently the words used to begin and end sessions, timing and tone of interpretations or manner in which bills are dispensed can be traced directly to supervisors or therapists. The emerging professional is undeniably significantly affected by his or her adult identifications. The relationship between the adult development process and mental-health education is discussed more completely in Chapter 15.

Hypothesis IV. The Fundamental Developmental Issues of Childhood Continue as Central Aspects of Adult Life but in Altered Form

If we begin to think of developmental issues in terms of the life cycle, it is possible to clarify the forms taken by such basic processes as separation–individuation and oedipal phenomena in various phases of life *rather than understand them only as significant events of childhood*. One of the few subjects that have been approached in this manner is the separation–individuation process, examined by three coordinated panels of the American Psychoanalytic Association.

Through the study of young children, Mahler, Pine, and Bergman (1975) have described the process by which the human infant gradually emerges as a separate, distinct being, aware of its own existence and nature and of its relationship to others. The name given by Mahler to this process, which is largely determined by the relationship between mother and child during the first three years of life, is the separation–individuation process.

In one of the panels of the American Psychoanalytic Association, Mahler (Winestine, 1973) described separation–individuation as a lifelong process because of the inherent threat of loss in every stage of independence. The *absolute* dependence on the mother which is characteristic of infancy becomes a *relative* dependence in later life. Spiegel defined an aspect of maturity, a goal only partially realized even in the healthy adult, as "objective independence" (Marcus, 1973, p. 163); namely, the recognition of the object ("object" is synonomous with "person") in its own right without reference to the self, the recognition that both self and loved one have independence. What Spiegel is describing, we believe, it the *transformation* of an infantile theme into an adult one. Other theorists (Steinschein, 1973) speak of the adult need to redefine oneself and relationships to significant people at such critical, affect-laden junctures as marriage, parenthood, grandparenthood, the climacteric, retirement, and senescence.

The Oedipal Complex

By "oedipal complex" we mean the grouping of instinctual wishes and fears toward the parents universally found at the height of the phallic phase, ages three to six. "During this period the child strives in a limited way for sexual union with the parent of the opposite sex and the death or disappearance of the parent of the same sex " (Moore & Fine, 1968, p. 66). The continuation of the oedipal complex into adulthood is not a new idea. Freud (1924) spoke of it in *The Dissolution of the Oedipal Complex*, as did Pearson (1958), Benedek (1975), and others, but little has been written about oedipal phenomena as central, continuing factors in normal adult development. One exception is in the article by Rangell (1953):

> The oedipal complex has a continuous and dynamic line of development, from its earliest origin through various phases in the life of man, and the described phenomena are but stages in the continual moving stream. By no means is it an event which plays a tumultuous but short-lived role limited to the phallic scene of the play of life, but it is rather a constantly reappearing character which comes across the stage in new and changing ways progressing with the ages of man. (p. 13)

There is much to describe regarding oedipal phenomena in the normal adult. Each parent reacts to the budding sexuality of adolescent children with at least occasional overrestriction or seductiveness. Aware of the muting of sexual prowess in midlife and unconsciously jealous of the adolescent's abundant future, the parent retaliates against his offspring (Pearson, 1958). Competitiveness and envy of girl friends or boy friends, fiancés and fiancées, and eventually husbands and wives of grown children provide ample evidence of the triangular relationships that exist among parents, children, and children's spouses. Fathers' protectiveness of their daughters' virtue and encouragement of their sons' lack of it, and mother-in-laws' almost universal tendency to compete for their children are all-too-obvious evidence of the nature of adult oedipal phenomena.

These oedipal phenomena are responded to by the normal adult with capabilities that make the experience qualitatively different from that of the child. The following factors illustrate this point: (1) The adult body is sexually mature and, unlike the child's, has the capacity for release through foreplay and intercourse. An intimate, loving heterosexual relationship provides a mechanism for working through unresolved sexual conflicts that are stimulated by interactions with oedi-pal-age, adolescent, and young-adult offspring (Kernberg, 1974). (2) The mature psychic apparatus of the adult provides means for muting, modulating, and expressing oedipal feelings. The integrated conscience of the adult, absent in the oedipal child, will not tolerate the direct ex-pression of incestual fantasies toward one's children. Secondly, the adult capacities to reason, use judgment, and assess consequences mit-igate against blatant behavioral and verbal expression of oedipal wishes as are seen in the young child. Nor should we forget the increased ca-pacity for the more acceptable sublimation of these feelings afforded by such adult options as work and creativity. (3) Another avenue available to the adult for the expression of oedipal feelings is relationships with friends and work associates, who also are available for ventilation of the stresses incumbent in parenthood. The young child, fairly well con-fined to the nuclear family and unable independently to form meaning-ful relationships outside of it, is trapped by circumstance and his im-maturity.

Hypothesis V. The Developmental Processes in Adulthood Are Influenced by the Adult Past as Well as the Childhood Past

We would like to expand the use of the genetic approach (refer-ence to the past) to place more importance on adult experience. When we use the term "genetic" we usually refer to the childhood past—for example, how the events of the oedipal phase determine the formation of a neurosis in our adult patient, or how the successful traversal of ad-olescence resulted in the uniqueness of adult-character formation (Blos, 1968).

But what of the young-adult past or the middle-age past? What part do they play in our understanding of normal and pathological adult behavior? In our more open-end concept of development, "ge-netic" takes on a longitudinal dimension, incorporating new experi-ences that occur at each developmental phase throughout life. These more recent experiences undoubtedly relate to and are influenced by the events of childhood, but cannot be fully explained by them.

> L. was 38 when he entered treatment for "an absence of feeling and impotence." He was highly successful and creative in his business but unable to sustain any degree of sexual or emotional closeness with his wife of many years. There were numerous infantile experiences which

readily explained his behavior: a seductive mother, a sexually inhibited, distant father who preached the evils of sex, and who was seated at his bedside when he awoke at age five from a circumcision for which he was not prepared.

His sexual development was hampered throughout adolescence but in his twenties he was able to marry, father a child, and achieve academically. Sexual performance gradually improved throughout the early years of his marriage, indicating some mastery of his infantile sexual conflicts through adult sexual experience, when suddenly at age 30 a mass was discovered on his testicle. The resulting surgery and radiation for his testicular cancer had a profound effect upon his future sexual and emotional development. Years of sexual frustration and emotional withdrawal followed. His repressed rage at the doctors for sterilizing him, his inability to mourn the loss of his procreative capacity, and his use of work and creativity to avoid further close emotional and sexual contact with his wife were constant themes in the therapy.

The connection between these adult factors and childhood experiences such as the circumcision and great reliance on his intelligence to attract his mother and appease his literary father all eventually became clear, but were not sufficient in themselves to remove the emotional and sexual blocks to his adult fulfillment.

The analysis of the effect of the cancer on his *adult* aspirations—his wish to father another child, the loss of the sexual intimacy with his wife which was developing spontaneously at the time, and the seeming inability to feel any emotion because of an unrecognized fear of death—was the key to an empathetic, therapeutic alliance which resulted in an exploration of both infantile and adult determinants of his behavior and a resolution of his problems. To this man the *adult* past was infinitely more important than the infantile past, and for the therapist thinking in adult-developmental terms, understanding the adult past was the key to successful treatment.

The male climacteric is another example of the effect of adult experience on the developmental process. As described by Benedek and Maranon (1954), the typical male response to the climacteric is fantasized or actual attempts to deny the slow but inevitable sexual decline. The response to this process is not based solely on infantile factors, although they are obviously of great importance. Adult experience with intimacy is also an important determinant of the response. For example, a man of 55, fortunate enough to have a successful marriage in which there is a close sense of sharing with a trusted and loving wife, may be able to accept the inevitable more gracefully because sexual functioning is only one component of their mutually satisfying relationship. The sharing of interests and values in a strong marriage is a powerful resource, unavailable in childhood, for coping with developmental crises. So either in emotional crises or in the normal developmental experiences of adulthood the recent adult past has profound importance.

Hypothesis VI. Development in Adulthood, as in Childhood, Is Deeply Influenced by the Body and Physical Change

Freud (1915a) placed great emphasis on the influence of the body in mental development. For example, the concept of erogenous zones is a cornerstone of Freudian theory. We refer to oral, anal, and phallic zones, circumscribed areas of heightened bodily sensations which are partially responsible for mental development in childhood. Critics describe this theory as speculative and unsubstantiated, and although it is easily defended on clinical and observational grounds, only rarely is reference made to *biological* data. The theory describes, somewhat vaguely, a cephalo-caudal progression of neurological maturation which during the anal phase, for example, leads to myelinization of the lower extremities and the resultant capacity for locomotion and sphincter control. But, in the main, existing biological data on physical maturation have not been integrated with psychodynamic thought, and the literature is practically devoid of articles on the relationship between the biochemical and hormonal events of childhood and normal development.

Integration of mind and body is most clearly described in the theory of adolescence. The profound biological upheaval of puberty renders much existing mental organization inadequate and requires a reworking of psychic structure with basic alterations in the mental apparatus. A number of years are required to integrate these changes and again achieve a balanced relationship between mind and body.

For the adult years, a span much longer than childhood, we have no defined theory of mind–body relationship until the obvious occurrence of the climacteric; then biological variables are again considered (Benedek & Maranon, 1954). Even Erikson (1963), who refers to bodily zones and modes through adolescence, speaks of adulthood only in terms of abstract concepts such as "intimacy," "generativity," and "stagnation."

What are the normal biological and maturational events of adulthood, and how would awareness of them help us achieve a more complete understanding of mental development? Recent research is changing our concepts of brain functioning and may have important implications for analytic theory.

In *Instincts and Their Vicissitudes,* Freud (1915a) elaborated the concept of instincts to describe the influence of the body on the mind.

> If we now apply ourselves to considering mental life from a *biological* point of view, an "instinct" appears to us as a concept on the frontier between the mental and the somatic, as the physical representative of the stimuli originating from within the organism and reaching the mind, as a measure of the demand made upon the mind for work in consequence of its connection with the body. (pp. 121–122)

Freud did not feel that a detailed understanding of the biological process underlying the instinctual drives was necessary for his theory, and years later, Rapaport (1960) concurred:

> (a) The laws of functioning of the mental apparatus (i.e. the laws of behavioral regulation) can and must be investigated by a study of behavior (or if you prefer, molar behavior) without reference to molecular, physiological or neural processes; and (b) the relationships of the explanatory constructs derived from behavior to somatic processes must be kept vague at least as long as our knowledge of both types of process is meager, less psychological concepts (or even behaviors) be prematurely equated or tied to specific physiological processes. (p. 194)

In our opinion, by questioning the *relevance* of biological knowledge to psychological theory, such statements have inhibited efforts to integrate advances in biological research with theories of mental functioning and have impeded the development of integrated theory of mind–body interaction for the entire life cycle.

Neurological Factors

In most biological and psychological literature the adult body and brain are described either as structurally stable or as undergoing gradual physiological retrogression and loss. The *loss phenomenon* dominates—loss of physical prowess, loss of neurons, loss of intelligence. For example, Soddy (1967) reported that central-nervous-system decline begins in the middle twenties with a gradual diminution in brain weight, followed in the early thirties by a decrease in total lipids, which indicate brain maturity. Wechsler (1941) described a similar pattern for intellectual capacity:

> . . . intellectual ability after reaching a maximum at 20–25 does not continue unaltered for any length of time but starts trailing off immediately thereaf-

ter. Beginning at age 30, the rate of decline maintains almost a constant
slope. Intellectual decline follows the same general decline as does physical
ability. (p. 46)

Perhaps it is the anxious response to growing old and the increased adult preoccupation with personal time limitations and ap-
proaching death that give an inner sense of conviction to such findings
and result in resistance to further exploration of the developmental
processes of adulthood. After all, it is the adult who must study the
adult, just as he has studied the child, even though a concentration on
the second half of the life cycle may stir up personal apprehension and
anxiety.

Recent neurological studies on normal biological processes in the
mature brain seem to contradict the earlier studies just mentioned.
Mechanisms have been described for the reorganization of existing
neurological structure and for the possibility of *new growth* in the mature brain stimulated in part by mental activity. For example, Pribram
(1971) asks why the problem of the biology of memory, evidence that
experience produces permanent modification in neural tissues, proved
so difficult? In other parts of the body, when a *structure changes in a
healthy way over time*, growth and development of tissues occurs. But in
the brain, the number of neurons does not increase after an initial period following birth. Thus, the paradox is that nearly all behavioral development and learning seems to occur in the absence of obvious evidence of neural growth.

Pribram describes three responses to this paradox. The first attempts to establish that some other form of *neural growth* occurs as a
function of experience. The second involves the proliferation of *neuroglia*, the nonneural elements of neural tissues that increase in quantity
over the lifetime of an individual. The third alternative suggests that
important modifications take place within *chemical* storage processes in
the brain.

Pribram's main ideas related to these three possibilities can be
summarized as follows:

Neural Growth. Growth cones are the means by which neurons
grow, but usually there is not enough extracellular space in the central
nervous system to permit new neural growth. However, the situation
changes when the brain is injured. In gross injury the routine reaction
of the brain is to destroy the injured parts and to liquefy them, leaving
a hole or cyst. Rose, Malis, and Baker (1961) used cyclotron radiation to

produce minute lesions which created space between nerve fibers and resulted in a thickening of surrounding fibers, indicating that growth had taken place. Pribram (1971) similarly concluded that " . . . fibers' growth is possible in the mature brain if the circumstances for growth are favorable" (p. 21).

Neural growth has been produced in other ways as well. In experiments with rats, stimulation by play and problem solving resulted in thickening of the cortex. Histological analysis revealed an increase in the number of branchings of basal dendrites and the distension of dendritic spines (the small, hairlike protrusions on the dendrites which are presumed to be active, functional sites). There were also a large increase in nonneural cells (glia) and an actual decrease in numbers of neurons.

The Role of Neuroglia. Glia, which originates from the same embryonic tissue as nerve cells, is known to provide nutrient support to neurons and may guide the direction of growth cones and alter the activity of neural aggregates which are embedded in them. Thus it may be possible to attribute to glia, usually thought of as strictly supportive tissue, an important function as a growth stimulator and producer.

Chemical Modification. Chemical alteration, in any of several forms, may hold the key to brain modification in the absence of neuronal change. The first such possibility described by Pribram (1971) involves the role of glia and neurons in memory mechanisms through RNA and DNA production. "There appears to be no question that RNA production is somehow involved when nerves are stimulated physiologically or when the organism performs a task" (p. 38). The synthesis of protein macromolecules referred to by Sjostrand (1969) provides a second possible biochemical base for modification; a third relates to the functioning of chemical neurotransmitters, increasingly referred to as "brain hormones," which may be stored and released in altered quantities at different times in life and under changing conditions of stimulation.

Thus, neural modifiability in the mature brain appears to be multidetermined. The presence of multiple mechanisms for the reorganization of neural structures requires the abandoning of any conception of the brain as a static, slowly decaying organ. Growth processes, apparently in response to environmental and internal stimulation, are also present and must be accounted for in our theory.

For example, accepted theory (Peller, 1954; Waelder, 1933) holds that play is an attempt to deal with the continuous traumatic stimulation which is the natural condition of the child. The immature mind of the child cannot comfortably handle the stimulation which continually impinges on it from within and without. With increased development the growing child, and certainly the emerging adult, is able to deal more comfortably with routine stimuli and there is no longer the nearly constant need to play.

Thus, the play of children (as well as other forms of mental activity) may (if evidence from animal studies is applicable) produce an organic effect, the thickening of the cortex, indicating increased neural interconnections. The result could be the development of a neural and mental organization capable of dealing with traumatic stimulation. Play would become a part of a mental-neural interaction that promotes cortical development, thus providing the neurological underpinning for emerging mental mechanisms. In the adult, it is now well established by 40-year longitudinal studies (Jarvik, Eisdofer, & Blum, 1973) that intelligence, as measured by psychological testing, continues to *increase* through the middle adult years into the seventh and eighth decades. We explain the evolution of this important capacity by hypothesizing that adult mental activity, in the form of work, play, and fantasy, stimulates the formation of increased neuronal interconnections which form the biological basis for the continual increase in IQ throughout the adult years. These examples from childhood and adulthood suggest a new function for the mind: that is, the stimulation of continual biological change in the brain by bringing together external and internal stimuli.

These ideas only hint at work that needs to be done to integrate the new brain biology and psychodynamic theory. A more detailed review of the most recent research on the body and brain is presented in Chapter 6.

Hypothesis VII. A Central, Phase-specific Theme of Adult Development Is the Normative Crisis Precipitated by the Recognition and Acceptance of the Finiteness of Time and the Inevitability of Personal Death

Each developmental phase from infancy to healthy adulthood "can be shown to contain disturbing concomitants which are characteristic," wrote Anna Freud (1976). In the child some of these are diffuse distress states in infancy, accident proneness in the toddler, and clinging and whininess during the separation–individuation process. In our clinical experience the most striking "disturbing concomitants" in midlife are associated with the increased awareness of time limitation and death. This awareness is an integral and essential part of the developmental process because it stimulates further development and integration as well as regression.

Freud (1915b) noted that "we show an unmistakable tendency to put death to one side, to eliminate it from life." There is nothing instinctual in us, he said, which responds to a belief in death. In the timelessness of the unconscious we are convinced of our immortality. The first half of life is characterized by a tendency to deny the inevitability of personal death. In childhood and adolescence the denial is bolstered by the immaturity of the psychic apparatus, limited awareness and understanding of the concept of time, and the progressive physical and psychological forces that characterize childhood development. There is little in the anabolic thrust of the developmental process to indicate a personal end.

The first crack in the armor appears to come in late adolescence when intrapsychic loss is felt keenly and normally experienced through a loosening of ties to the parents. A sense of history develops with a recognition of a personal past, present, and future (Seton, 1974). But the dawning recognition is quickly defended against by the optimism and idealism of the young adult—an attempt, says Jacques (1965) to deny the "two fundamental features of human life—the inevitableness of eventual death, and the existence of hate and destructive impulses inside each person" (p. 505). Gradually the belief in the inherent goodness of man, a central characteristic of the idealism of youth, is replaced by "a more contemplative pessimism" (p. 504) as awareness of the power of hate and destructive forces which contribute to man's misery, tragedy, and death increases.

But in midlife—the fourth, fifth, and sixth decades of life—the defensive maneuvers alter and the normal adult meets with his own finiteness as he recognizes and accepts the signs that confront him from every side: (1) physical signs of aging appear and multiply—grey hair, wrinkles, slowing of reflexes, moderation of sexual drive, menopause and male climacteric. (2) The death of parents, friends, and contemporaries must be dealt with. The death of the parents in particular undercuts the sense of unending continuance and security provided in childhood by the good-enough parent. One is left alone with the recognition that one will die as one's parents did. The death of a parent is a major change in an adult's life, bringing with it opportunity for profound internal reorganization, including increased separation–individuation, further resolution of the oedipal complex, and a new or altered relationship with the remaining parent. (3) The maturing of one's own children into adulthood shatters the sense of perpetual youth because identification of the childhood self with young children is no longer possible, as they become as big as, bigger than, and independent of oneself. (4) It becomes clear that not all one's life's ambitions and goals will be realized and that there is not enough time remaining to achieve new ones to equal importance.

The adult at midlife is at a critical juncture on the developmental continuum. And as at all such junctures, there is the potential for progression or regression. We feel there is some evidence of normal regression in all adults. The "disturbing concomitants" of this developmental crisis take many forms but include excessive, inappropriate physical activity or inadequate attention to bodily needs; competitiveness and envy of adolescent and young-adult children; abandonment or neglect of aging parents; or inappropriate sexual activity such as affairs with much younger men or women.

Pathological responses can take the form of the abandonment of formerly stable marriages and productive careers in a frenzied attempt to begin anew, to reverse the passage of time.

> A productive, athletic man of 40, proud of his physical ability, developed an acute anxiety attack in response to minor surgery. He verbalized that his life was over, that his youth was lost. In a brief period of time he began an affair with a much younger woman, quarreled with his bewildered teen-age children, abandoned his outstandingly successful career, and became involved in strange and exotic theories and practices.

But pathology is not the main subject of this book, and we believe that too little attention has been paid to the stimulus to *forward* development and progression that is provided by this normative crisis of midlife. Confronting the quintessential adult-human experience can lead to ego functioning and integration of the highest order and produce the profoundest awareness of what it means to be human.

How does this stimulus work? The role of frustration as a stimulus to growth and development in childhood is a well-established concept. For example, parental frustration of oral drives through weaning, anal impulses through toilet training, and of oedipal impulses through modesty and a refusal to respond to the seductive wishes of the child all lead to mastery of the impulses involved and permit developmental progression. In the adult there are no frustrating parents to stimulate growth. But there is a mature mind capable of tolerating the frustration generated by the recognition that some impulses may not be gratified the way they were in earlier stages of development and others will not be gratified at all. Eventually the ultimate frustration, death, will result in the loss of all gratification.

Gradually the adult personality, stimulated by the awareness of time limitation and personal death, may reorganize along a positive line. For example: (1) Increased awareness of physical retrogression can lead to a redefinition of body image and act as a stimulus to developing new physical and nonphysical means of gratification appropriate to a realistic level of physical competence. (2) The sense of time limitation can be perceived as a stimulus to redefine goals and channel existing energy and resources into *obtainable* objectives that gratify the self and loved ones. (3) The conscience may be affected by the deaths of parents (Steinschein, 1973) and by increased demands for gratification of impulses that were held in check when time was thought to be plentiful. The effect of these midlife issues on psychic structure has barely been studied and is a fertile field for further investigation.

And what of the narcissistic investment in the self, a self no longer seen as omnipotent and everlasting? If we use Eriksonian psychology to approach this subject we might conclude that the failure to redefine the self leads to despair in old age rather than ego integrity. To quote Erikson (1963):

> It is a post-narcissistic love of the human ego—not of the self—as an experience which conveys some world order and spiritual sense . . . the acceptance of one's one and only life cycle as something that has to be . . . it is a comradeship with the ordering ways of distant times and different pursuits. (p. 268)

The failure to achieve this state of integration (the stimulus for which, we believe, is provided in the manner just described) leads to a magnified despair and fear of death in old age rather than to acceptance of the eventual loss of the self.

SUMMARY

The developmental framework, when applied to adulthood, emphasizes the continuing evolution of the personality at five or 50 and "focuses on the formation of psychic structure in process and under-scores the continuity of normal and pathologic outcomes" (Conference on Psychoanalytic Education and Research, 1974, p. 14). Many of the events we have discussed here are experiences unique to the adult and outside the realm of the child. Their uniqueness and developmental significance need to be better accounted for in psychodynamic theory.

Confrontation with each adult-developmental task or crisis pro-duced basic change in the life of each individual. To quote Bibring (1959):

> We find them as developmental phenomena at points of no return be-tween one phase and the next when decisive changes deprive former cen-tral needs and modes of living of their significance forcing the acceptance of highly charged new goals and functions. (p. 119)

One purpose of this chapter has been to demonstrate that such de-velopmental turning points of no return are not limited to childhood but occur throughout the life cycle.

References

Benedek, T. Parenthood as a developmental phase. *Psychoanalytic Quarterly*, 1950, *19*, 1.

Benedek, T. Depression during the life cycle. In E. J. Anthony & T. Benedek (Eds.), *De-pression and human existence*. Boston: Little, Brown, 1975.

Benedek, T., & Maranon, G. The climacteric. In A. M. Karch (Ed.), *Men: The variety and meaning of the sexual experience*. New York: Dell, 1954.

Bibring, G. Some considerations of the psychological processes in pregnancy. *Psychoana-lytic Study of the Child*, 1959, 14, *113–121*.

Binstock, W. On the two forms of intimacy. *Journal of the American Psychoanalytical Associa-tion*, 1973, 22, 743.

Blos, P. Character formation in adolescence. *Psychoanalytic Study of the Child*, 1968, 23, 245.

Conference on Psychoanalytic Education and Research. Commission IX, "Child Anal-ysis." New York: American Psychoanalytic Association, 1974.

Eissler, K. On possible effects of aging on the practice of psychoanalysis: An essay. *Jour-nal of the Philadelphia Association for Psychoanalysis*, 1975, *11*, 139.

Erikson, E. H. *Childhood and society* (2nd ed.). New York: W. W. Norton, 1963.

Erikson, E. H. *Dimensions of a new identity: Jefferson lectures*. New York: W. W. Norton, 1974.

Freud, A. Psychopathology seen against the background of normal development. *British Journal of Psychiatry*, 1976, *129*, 201.

Freud, A., Nagera, H., & Freud, E. Metapsychological assessment of the adult personal-ity. *Psychoanalytic Study of the Child*, 1965, 29, 9.

Freud, S. The interpretation of dreams. Standard edition 4:1. London: Hogarth Press, 1900.

Freud, S. Three essays on the theory of sexuality. Standard edition 7:125. London: Hogarth Press, 1905.

Freud, S. The case of little Hans. Standard edition 10:3. London: Hogarth Press, 1909.

Freud, S. *Instincts and their vicissitudes*. Standard edition 14:109. London: Hogarth Press, 1915. (a)

Freud, S. *Thoughts for the times on war and death*. Standard edition 14:273. London: Hogarth Press, 1915. (b)

Freud, S. *The dissolution of the Oedipus complex*. Standard edition 19:173. London: Hogarth Press, 1924.

Gould, R. L. *Transformations: Growth and change in adult life*. New York: Simon & Schuster, 1978.

Hartmann, H. *Ego psychology and the problem of adaptation*. New York: International Universities Press, 1958. (Originally published, 1939.)

Jacques, E. Death and the mid-life crisis. *International Journal of Psycho-Analysis*, 1965, *46*, 602.

Jarvik, L. J., Eisdofer, C., & Blum, J. E. *Intellectual functioning in adults*. New York: Springer, 1973.

Kernberg, O. Mature love: Prerequisites and characteristics. *Journal of the American Psychoanalytic Association*, 1974, *22*, 743.

Levinson, D. J., Darrow, C. N., Klein, E. B., Levinson, M. H., & McKee, B. *The seasons of a man's life*. New York: Alfred A. Knopf, 1978.

Mahler, M., Pine, F., & Bergman, A. *The psychological birth of the human infant*. New York: Basic Books, 1975.

Marcus, I. (Reporter). The experience of separation–individuation . . . through the course of life: Adolescence and maturity (Panel report). *Journal of the American Psychoanalytic Association*, 1973, *21*, 155.

Moore, B., & Fine, B. *A glossary of psychoanalytic terms and concepts*. New York: American Psychoanalytic Association, 1968.

Parens, H. (Reporter) Parenthood as a developmental phase. In *Panel reports*. *Journal of the American Psychoanalytic Association*, 1975, *23*, 154–165.

Pearson, G. *Adolescence and the conflict of generations*. New York: W. W. Norton, 1958.

Peller, L. Libidinal phases, ego development and play. *Psychoanalytic Study of the Child*, 1954, *9*, 178–198.

Pribram, K. *Languages of the brain: Experimental paradoxes and principles in neuropsychology*. Englewood Cliffs, N.J.: Prentice-Hall, 1971, pp. 3–47.

Rangell, L. The role of the parent in the Oedipus complex. *Bulletin of the Menninger Clinic*, 1953, *19*, 9.

Rapaport D. On the psychoanalytic theory of motivation. In M. R. Jones (Ed.), *Nebraska Symposium on Motivation*. Lincoln: University of Nebraska Press, 1960, pp. 173–247.

Rose, J., Malis, L., & Baker C. Neural growth in the cerebral cortex after lesions produced by monoenergetic denterous. In W. A. Rosenblith (Ed.), *Sensory communication*. New York: Wiley, 1961, pp. 279–301.

Seton, P. The psychotemporal adaptation of late adolescence. *Journal of the American Psychoanalytic Association*, 1974, *22*, 795.

Shane, M. A rationale for teaching analytic technique based on a developmental orientation and approach. *International Journal of Psycho-Analysis*, 1977, *58*, 95.

Sjostrand, F. The molecular structure of membranes. In S. Bogoch (Ed.), *The future of the brain sciences*. New York: Plenum Press, 1969, pp. 117–157.

Soddy, K. *Men in middle age*. New York: J. B. Lippincott, 1967.

Spitz, R. *The first year of life*. New York: International Universities Press, 1965.

Steinschein, I. (Reporter). The experience of separation-individuation . . . through the course of life: Maturity, senescence, and sociological implications (Panel report). *Journal of the American Psychoanalytic Association*, 1973, *21*, 633.

Vaillant, G. *Adaptation to life*. Boston: Little, Brown, 1977.

Waelder, R. The psychoanalytic theory of play. *Psychoanalytic Quarterly*, 1933, 2, 208.

Wechsler, D. Intellectual changes with age. *Mental Health in Later Maturity*, Supp. 168, Federal Security Agency, United States Public Health Service, 1941, pp. 43–52.

Winestine, M. (Reporter). The experience of separation-individuation . . . through the course of life: Infancy and childhood (Panel report). *Journal of the American Psychoanalytic Association*, 1973, 21, 135.

5

Narcissism in the Adult Development of the Self

In this chapter, building on the work of Kernberg (1977), Kohut (1971), Loewald (1960), Saperstein and Gaines (1973), and other authors, we explore the nature of the adult self, concentrating on a description of its emergence and characteristics, and the narcissistic issues that underlie its development. By narcissism we mean

> a concentration of psychological interest upon the self . . . .Under normal circumstances, people's interests are divided between a concern for themselves (narcissism) and for the world of things and people around them (object love). (Moore & Fine, 1968, p. 62)

Kohut (1977), in describing the development of psychoanalysis, urged the addition of a concept of the self because, like Lichtenberg (1975), he felt that our understanding of the complexities of the mind would be aided by new frames of reference. However, the self as a specific concept has been difficult to integrate with existing psychodynamic theory. Rosenblatt and Thickstun (1977) wrote:

> The self, which currently occupies a position within standard structural theory somewhere between the ego and limbo, can be conceptualized as the superordinate system, or the organism itself, encompassing *all* of the systems operating within the organism. This concept of the self in the sense of the person must, however, be distinguished from the experimental concept of *self as agent*, which involves awareness of choice, decision, and reflective awareness of oneself as the agent of such choice or decision. (p. 300)

The basis for this chapter is an article by the authors entitled "Authenticity and Narcissism in the Adult Development of the Self" which was published in the *Annual of Psychoanalysis*, 1980, 8.

Jacobson (1965) was one of the first authors to write systematically about the self concept. In a statement of considerable descriptive value she said:

> By a realistic image of the self, we mean first of all, one that correctly mirrors the state and the characteristics, the potentialities and abilities, the assets and the limits of our bodily and mental self: on the one hand, of our appearance, our anatomy, and our physiology; on the other hand, of our ego, our conscious and preconscious feelings and thoughts, wishes, impulses, and attitudes toward our physical and mental functions and behavior. (p. 22)

Jacobson quotes Kramer (1955), who states that all of the above will have corresponding psychic representations, and that a concept of their sum total will develop, that is, "an awareness of the self as a differentiated but organized entity which is separate and distinct from one's environment" (p. 47). Jacobson also found Lichtenstein's (1961) description of self useful: "the self has the capacity to remain the same in the midst of change" (p. 193).

Saperstein and Gaines (1973) describe the confusion in the literature over the use of the term "ego" to refer to the personal self. They feel that "it is important to use the term 'personal self' to refer to the individual's sense of self as agent, or self as 'I'—the experiential awareness of his uniqueness, as a creator of meanings" (p. 415). The concept of self refers to the sense of the person's "I" as a free agent in the creation of what is meaningful to him. They refer the final determination of action to the self and suggest the usefulness of conceiving an overall, integrative self that mediates the interaction of the person as a whole with his environment. We are in essential agreement with Saperstein and Gaines's concepts and will utilize them in our description of the self in adulthood.

NARCISSISM AND THE ADULT SELF

Relatively little has been written about the vicissitudes of narcissism throughout the life cycle. Lichtenberg (1975), in describing the sense of self in childhood, has organized three lines of development relating narcissistic issues to the sense of self: (1) self-images based on body experiences associated with instinctual need satisfactions; (2) self-images that emerge as entities having discrete differentiation from others; and (3) self-images that by virtue of idealization retain a sense of grandiosity and omnipotence shared with an idealized person, such as mother. In describing how the self becomes cohesive, Lichtenberg writes of a lifelong "blending and balancing" (p. 470) of the above three clusters of self-images.

Eissler (1975) described a shifting with aging of narcissistic investments; Kernberg (1977) has suggested that normal narcissistic gratifications in adulthood increase self-esteem. Insofar as such gratification is closely linked with relationships to others, it strengthens them and their inner representations, and in the process shapes the adult self. The self is further modified by narcissistic gratifications that come from work, creativity, and "an internal build-up of the non-personal world of nature and things" (p. 7).

We plan to describe the relationship between the adult self and narcissism in detail, and we present the following basic concepts as an introduction to that discussion. Each individual must engage the narcissistic issues involved in the major developmental tasks of adulthood, and such issues are central to the development of the adult self. It is not enough to resolve the narcissistic issues of early life; adult life brings *new* ones into play. Forces that modify the adult self are fueled by narcissistic gratifications and disappointments in *adulthood*. We include in our use of the term "gratifications" the self-nurturing fantasy process which in the integrated person is closely related to reality and often leads to realistic action (similar to Kohut's "healthy narcissism"). We call this process in adulthood *healthy self-aggrandizement*. Narcissistic disappointments affect the evolution of self as differences between idealizations and realities become clear; for example, the differences between one's idealized infant and the real child who emerges with increasing clarity over time.

Narcissistic issues from earlier developmental phases obviously have a major effect on the evolution of the adult self. Just as the adolescent relied upon the accomplishments of latency to bolster him against the regressive and narcissistic injuries of adolescence, so the adult gains sustenance from the accomplishments of young adulthood and gratifications provided therefrom such as the attainment of heterosexual intimacy and career goals.

The Authentic Self

From the Greek *authentikos,* and from the French *authentes* which refers to "one who does things himself," "genuine," "real,"[1] we have chosen the word *authentic* to describe the mature adult self because the term conveys a sense of intrapsychic recognition that one is singular (separated psychologically from parents yet interdependent with important people in the present), and capable of making and accepting a realistic appraisal of life, including suffering, limitation, and personal death. Authenticity, therefore, includes the capacity to assess and accept what is real in both the external and inner world, regardless of the narcissistic injury involved.

We see the attainment of authenticity as a central, dynamic task of adulthood, possible in its fullest sense in adulthood because of the nature of the adult-developmental process. In the healthy adult this process includes normative, intrapsychic conflict involving opposing tendencies to unrealistically inflate or deflate the self. Gradually the narcissistic position of childhood in which the self is characterized as special, unique, and qualitatively superior to all others (Kohut's grandiose self) must be abandoned and replaced by an acceptance of the self as special but not unique, a part of the mosaic of humanity. With the muting of the quest for perfection in the self, in others, and in the external world—a concept rooted in the vicissitudes of the early mother-child dyad—comes gradual acceptance of the self as imperfect.

Authenticity includes the capacity to resist the sometimes powerful middle-age impulse to search regressively for more complete gratification (infantile perfection) as a defense against the loosening of intrapsychic ties to aging or dead parents and to operate alone (psychologically separated from them) within the limits imposed by an imperfect, partially gratifying, and sometimes hostile world. Initially a source of narcissistic injury, the recognition of these external and internal limitations gradually becomes a source of pleasure and strength as the self accepts and develops the capacity to act independently within the restrictions imposed by the human condition.

Implicit in this process is the *normal mourning* (Pollock, 1961) which accompanies the awareness of the loss of such earlier forms of gratification as the assertive independence and intense sexuality characteristic

---

[1] *Webster's New World Dictionary of the American Language,* 1975.

of adolescence, or opportunities that occur in young adulthood to make basic decisions about the future like the choice of spouse, career, or number of children. Mourning for the adolescent and young-adult past (as well as for the early-infantile past) leads to a gradual restructuring of the self with new awareness: "This is what I am." "These are the gratifications available to me."

This process of loss, mourning, working through and restructuring of the self stimulates an active search for new, age-appropriate mechanisms for obtaining gratification, as opposed to pathological forms of mourning, including incomplete grief and depression, which impede further development. In the psychic process involved in these changes the fantasized, idealized, or negatively distorted conceptions of life prevailing in childhood and young adulthood are diminished in power and importance.

An example of authenticity is contained in the following statement from a middle-aged man at the end of his therapy.

> I'm not young any more, but I'm getting old gracefully. I've come to know what's meaningful in life—people. Nothing else matters much. I have my wife, my friends, and my work. None of those things will last forever; neither will I, for that matter, my parents didn't; but for the first time in my life, I see how it all fits together, and I've accepted my lot.

BASIC INFLUENCES IN THE DEVELOPMENT OF THE ADULT SELF

Thus the evolution of the self in adulthood is a dynamic process, part of the lifelong shaping of identity. We believe that a number of factors, some unique to adult experience, build on the self constructed from earlier phases of life and develop it further. Some of the most important among them are: (1) the body, (2) object ties, (3) time and death, and (4) work, creativity, and mentorship.

The Body and the Adult Self

The profound influence of the body in early mental development has been extensively delineated in Freud's (1915) concept of erogenous zones and their sequential predominancy, and it is likewise well documented that a balanced relationship between mind and body in young adulthood is achieved only after several years of intense reworking of the immature psychic apparatus which proves inadequate to the biological upheaval at puberty. Biological factors in the relationship between psyche and soma remain relatively unattended to until the climacteric (Benedek & Maranon, 1954). Even Erikson (1963), although he writes about bodily zones and modes through adolescence, uses only such abstract words as "intimacy," "generativity," and "stagnation" to describe the issues of mind and body integration in adults.

Recent studies on normal biological processes in the mature body and brain may have important implications because they describe mechanisms that characterize the adult body as being in a state of dynamic flux and change. Although the retrogressive process becomes increasingly powerful with age, it is not the only one at work. Progressive forces, including the possibility of new growth in the mature brain, stimulated in part by mental activity, have been described (Pribram, 1971).

Although there has been some recognition that the aging body can be a source of narcissistic injury (Cath, 1962) and in some narcissistic patients result in regression, we would like to emphasize that the response to aging is a normative experience as well.

In the course of midlife development, we suggest a *normative conflict* between wishes to deny the aging process and acceptance of the loss of a youthful body. The resolution of this conflict leads to a reshaping of the body image and a more realistic appraisal of the middle-aged body, resulting in a heightened sense of appreciation of the pleasures the body can continue to provide if cared for properly through appropriate activities.

This conflict may emerge in midlife as a search for a new body. Some middle-aged persons feel an urgent "need" for inappropriate forms of plastic surgery, while others leave spouses in search of the young who have the "hard body feel." In these individuals the normal mourning for their young-adult bodies seems to be short-circuited, and instead of the resolution of a normative developmental conflict they attempt a *magical repair of their body image* through surgery or by attempting to fuse with or borrow another person's younger body.

Another, more pathological form of regression stimulated by changes in the adult body can be the sudden emergence, for the first time, of perversions. To be sure, earlier fixations exist in such individuals, but we believe that specifically adult factors, namely, change in midlife bodily appearance and sexual functioning, can act as powerful traumata to trigger regression and perverse behavior.

For the first time in his life, a professional man in his forties found himself drawn to public bathrooms where he tried to catch sight of other men's penises. This situation progressed to one of homosexual entrapment and arrest by the police. When he came to treatment, it emerged that he had been devastated by the loss of his youthful appearance and several episodes of impotence. His behavior was felt to be an attempt to deny normal aging and achieve a magical repair of the sense of inadequacy he felt in his body as a whole and his penis in particular.

A middle-aged woman came to treatment because of a strong urge to have a number of sexual partners other than her husband. She said it was "like being in an ice cream store; if you can have five flavors, why only one?" She verbalized a sense of urgency and a feeling that time was running out on her. Among a number of issues, a definite theme about bodily changes emerged. She had decided to have a hysterectomy but was terrified that loss of the capacity to have children would leave her "dried up, empty and old." In addition she expressed the wish that through her affairs the vital, nurturing penises of young men would arrest her aging process and be her fountain of youth.

Summarizing these responses to the narcissistic injury involved in bodily changes during adulthood, we find the following:

1. *Repairing the body:* actual attempts at repair including plastic surgery, dyeing hair, makeup, exercise, and diet.

2. *Finding a new body:* the search for a new body or parts of a new body through hetero- or homosexual relationships.

3. *Substituting for the body:* adult toys and hobbies such as bigger and better boats, houses, cars, and so on which are used symbolically to compensate for and repair the changes in the body.

With resolution and working through of the crisis involved in adult bodily change comes a sense of narcissistic pleasure that includes a more conflict-free sexuality. This continued developmental enhancement of sexual pleasure and intimacy becomes an important expression of the integrated, authentic adult self.

Self and Object in Adult Development

In a recent series of panels (Marcus, 1973; Steinschein, 1973; Winestine, 1973), the theme of the separation-individuation processes was extended beyond childhood and adolescence through maturity and senescence. Mahler (1973) concluded that

. . . the entire life cycle constitutes a more or less successful process of distancing from and introjection of the lost symbiotic mother, an external longing for the actual or fantasized ideal state of self, with the latter standing for

> a symbiotic fusion with the all-good symbiotic mother who was at one time
> part of the self in a blissful state of well-being. (p. 138)

Thus the quest for a clearer differentiation between self and others ends only with biological death. In addition to the major separation-individuation phases that occur in childhood and in adolescence, we observe significant *new* separation-individuation phenomena in the young-adult period (the third separation-individuation phase). As Erikson (1963) has stated, each adult phase can be understood to have its intrinsic tasks and goals, leading to sharper self-other differentiation and new aspects of identity. What follows is our description of the effect of relationships in adulthood upon the emerging adult self.

Shifting Object Ties

The healthy adult recognizes, as part of his authentic appraisal of reality, the central position of change in his life. A basic aspect of that change is the shifting nature of significant emotional relationships. Adult involvement with loved ones such as children, parents, colleagues, and friends is in constant realignment. These ties continue to shift in middle age—when healthy marriages deepen in significance (while others break up on the shoals of middle-age developmental issues); parents die or become dependent; children grow and leave; and friends increase in importance and in some instances leave or die themselves. As opposed to old age and in some respects to childhood as well, the task is to sort out, categorize, set priorities among relationships, and achieve a balance between internal pressures and external demands.

We feel that these shifting relationships are major stimuli which influence change in the self through an increasing process of psychological individuation. A major function of the authentic self is the continual reassessment of who one *is* in relationships as compared with who one was. The lessening of preoccupations with distant- or recent-past relationships and the forging of an identity based on current ones (some gratifying and some painful) are the essential ways in which the self is altered. For example, one *was* a child, an adolescent, a new spouse, an apprentice in work; whereas one *is* the supporter of aging parents, a parent/grandparent, an accomplished worker.

The Recognition of Interdependence

As a direct result of such adult individuation, individuals attain more significant appreciation of a basic characteristic of all human relations—interdependence.

Examples are the parents' need of the child as a confirmation of their sexuality and a vehicle for generativity, the reliance of spouses on each other in the sharing of joy and inevitable illness and suffering, and the reversal of roles between adult child and aging parent. Deeper understanding of this dimension of human need leads to a developing capacity for nonambivalent gratitude. In the authentic adult, unlike the child who takes, uses, controls, and dominates, further muting of the grandiose position of infancy propels the self toward deeper, more meaningful interactions. To illustrate we will focus on some of the most important ties—to parents, spouse, and children.

Parents and Grandparents

The separation-individuation process is enhanced in adult life by relationships to aging parents and grandparents. The increasing dependence and eventual death of parents undermines the naïve, infantile mental representations of the parents as omnipotent and increases recognition of the vulnerability and impermanence of the self as well as the parents. *In other words, infantile narcissism loses its power to defend against the awareness of death and the passage of time.* We agree with Kernberg (1977), who describes changes in attitudes toward death as occurring throughout the life cycle. Jacques (1965) has specifically described death awareness and anxiety during midlife crises, but that is too narrow a time frame for the entirety of the process.

Narcissistic issues also play a part in grandparent-parent-child interactions. Grandparental idealization of grandchildren serves several defensive purposes: (a) denial of the passage of time and of old age, (b) a chance for magical repair of one's own life through the grandchild, and (c) a denial of the imperfection of the self by selective identification with particular qualities in the grandchild. The healthy grandparent sees the falseness of this idealization but still enjoys the continuity that multigenerational ties bring. The recognition that death is final enhances appreciation of the limited ways in which the self lives on through one's creations and offspring.

The aging and death of parents and adult experiences such as sexual intimacy, parenthood, and the achievement of a work identity also change the self by producing basic alterations in the internal configuration of fundamental developmental issues of childhood which, in our opinion, continue in altered form as central aspects of adult life.

As an illustration, consider the changes that occur in adult oedipal representations of the parents. As an adult one has actually become a parent, and in a sense "won" the oedipal victory by obtaining many of the prerogatives wished for in childhood. The victory is hollow, however, since infantile gratifications cannot be enjoyed by an adult particularly in relation to aging or dead parents.

A normal developmental task of middle age, then, is dealing with this oedipal "victory" as the infantile wishes to dominate and replace the parents are realized. It is our contention that the aging and death of parents force a reworking of oedipal constructions just as surely as the biological upheaval of puberty. The alteration in the adult self is profound; the infantile oedipal construction is inappropriate to the *present*, and changes in internal representations of the parent alter the image of parent as competitor or lover, leading to a heightened sense of individuation and authenticity.

The Spouse

The adult separation-individuation process is centered in the marital relationship. A developmental task of late adolescence related to adult separation-individuation is the psychic construction of an *idealized, fantasized mate*. Rooted in early-childhood relationships with parents and the adolescent's experience with sexuality, this construction develops within the late-adolescent self as the result of the psychological separation from the parents during adolescence. With its formation, some of the narcissistic investment in the mental representations of the parents of childhood is transferred to the idealized-mate representation.

After marriage a continuous, painful process goes on within the self as the idealized-spouse representation is replaced by the real-spouse representation. As the real spouse is reacted to and internal-

Table V. *Transition from Idealized- to Real-Spouse Representation*

Initially	1. Separation from parents	3. Conflict between idealized-spouse and real-spouse representations
Later	2. Narcissistic transfer and construction of idealized-spouse representation	4. Gradual abandonment of idealized-spouse—more acceptance of real-spouse representation

ized, a second narcissistic transfer takes place from the idealized-spouse representation, which is diminished in importance but never completely abandoned, to the real-spouse representation. We suggest that this process occurs in every healthy marriage and is conflictual because the abandonment of the aggrandized, infantile images is painful and the real-spouse representation never approximates the idealized state. This gradual narcissistic transfer is a prerequisite to the emergence of mature love. Table V presents the above issues schematically.

With the approach of middle age, the aging of the spouse and the self becomes the major narcissistic issue in marriage. The narcissistic injury felt in the aging process, particularly in relation to sexual activity, is compensated by the intimacy of this now long-standing, gratifying relationship. Normative conflict is experienced between the pull toward youthful bodies and sexual reassurance and the realistic acceptance of the adult body and the internal body image. The development of the real-spouse representation greatly facilitates this process by enhancing real intimacy, thus diminishing the narcissistic sting of aging.

Summarizing this section, there are two major narcissistic, developmental aspects of normal marriage. One, which occurs in early marriage, is the gradual acceptance of the real spouse over the idealized, fantasized spouse and the second, which occurs in middle age, is the acceptance of aging in the spouse. Both of these tasks are gradual, painful processes which, if mastered, facilitate the continued growth of the marriage and of the self.

We suggest that the appreciation and valuing of long-standing relationships, in contrast to the more youthful gratifications of the body and nonrelationship sex, is characteristic of the adult self and a major developmental step of midlife.

Children

Child rearing is another potential source of adult narcissistic gratification and disappointment. The vicissitudes of raising children powerfully affect feelings of self-worth and competence.

Parental gratifications and disappointments exist at each stage of a child's development, but probably peak in the child's adolescence. The healthy parent is gratified by the push toward independence of the adolescent instead of experiencing the loss of the child exclusively as a drain or injury. Through identification the parents attempt to reexperience and work through the disappointments and ambitions of their own youth.

> A patient ruminated about his adolescent son's continual athletic victories over him. Finally he expressed it this way: "Actually, when I think about it, I feel some pleasure, too. In some ways he's like an extension of me, and even though I can't do it any more the way I used to, he can, and he is my son."

Narcissistic experiences are a major influence on the quality of interaction with the child. The healthy parent, for the most part, quietly accepts the child's emerging identity and does not excessively "puff up" or "put down" his offspring. Rather, there is a steering toward a realistic self which is part of the parenting process. However, when children are related to as extensions of the self, the tendency to inflate unrealistically or deflate the child can be more pronounced.

> A patient remembered her mother's excessive praise for sweeping off the porch of her grandparents' house when she was a child. The patient in adult life expressed resentment over the mother's overblown and unrealistic praise: "I now see that she didn't do me any favor by puffing me up like that, nobody else thought I was so great." This patient is now putting a grandiose or overvalued self in perspective.

> Deflation of self by a parent was experienced by another patient who remembered days of adolescent glory on the football field. This patient's mother continually responded to athletic triumphs with statements like, "Don't let it go to your head," "It's really not that important," or "The important thing is you didn't get hurt." For the adolescent the athletic victories were a once-in-a-lifetime experience that was being devalued, leading to puzzling and confusing feelings.

There is an analogy between the parent's tendencies to overvalue or deflate as opposed to quiet, even acceptance of the child's emerging self and the narcissistic interaction between therapist and patient, for this relationship is essentially similar to the healthy parenting situation—a quiet, even acceptance of the patient's thoughts and feelings as therapy proceeds. Interpretations and silence can be experienced as critical deflations; excessive verbalizations and supportive praise can be felt as overvaluations.

Further Acceptance of Sexual Differences

Adult relationships affect not only separation-individuation but other aspects of development as well. One example which also illustrates the elaboration of infantile sexual themes in adulthood is the further acceptance of the female as different, not castrated or defective.

The attempt to understand and accept the sexual difference between male and female is a lifelong process beginning early in life and continuing throughout childhood. However, full acceptance and integration is only possible in adulthood because major adult experiences add new elements to the understanding of sexuality:

1. Repeated experiences with sexuality and intimacy lead to a thorough understanding of the *complementary differences* of the male and female genitalia through repeated sexual exploration of one's body and the genitals of the opposite sex. We have treated several neurotic men and women, most of them married and sexually active, in whom the capacity to look at, touch, and think about the partner's genitals was markedly inhibited. The gradual resolution of infantile and adult sexual problems allowed us to observe the developmental working through and integration of the complementary nature of the male and female genitals in subsequent sexual experience.

2. The experience of parenthood sharpens the sexual identity of a man and woman by underscoring their interdependence for procreation, thus validating the necessity for male and female genitalia. The experience of having produced an offspring with genitalia of either sex is another stimulus to this reworking and integration because of the powerful narcissistic investment of the parents in their child.

3. The experience of parenthood forces a reworking of earlier sexual attitudes as infantile sexuality is again engaged through the child at each developmental phase but from the vantage point of adult experience.

4. As previously mentioned, the changing relations to aging and dying parents produce a further resolution of the oedipal aspects of sexuality.

5. The change in the nature of sexual capacity produced by physical aging (such as menopause) produces a normative crisis that forces the subject of sexuality upon the self. The healthy adult who shares this experience with a loving sexual partner has the opportunity to integrate further aspects of sexual identity from a new perspective.

Time, Narcissism, and Authenticity

The normal middle-aged person is keenly aware of the limited amount of time in the future compared to the past. In our opinion, this recognition of time limitation and the inevitability of personal death is a major psychic organizer of the adult self. The forces that produce this dynamic focus are many, for the most part fairly obvious—the aging of the body, death of parents and friends, growth of children into adolescence and adulthood, and intrapsychic lengthening of the personal past and loosening of ties to the infantile introjects.

We are not talking of a psychopathological preoccupation with aging and death, but of the internal and external temporal stimuli that constantly impinge on the healthy adult self, directing attention to thoughts of time. The engagement of this developmental task of assessing one's past, present, and future is, we feel, a little-understood, *positive* developmental stimulus which has a profound effect on the adult self.

Time sense in childhood and adolescence is gratifying because time seems to exist in unlimited quantity. But by midlife time sense becomes a source of pain with the recognition that there is not enough left to gratify all wishes or redo unhappy aspects of the past.

For the healthy person this realization is cushioned by what we call the "gratifying past": those memories of childhood and young adulthood that are pleasurable and give the sense that one's life has been "good enough." This *middle-age nostalgia* is clearly a narcissistic defense against the growing awareness of time limitation; the narcissistic aspect is suggested by the warm feelings of timelessness, continuity, fusion, and gratification which accompany the nostalgia. Here is the repository (within the adult self) of the relationship with the good-enough mother, added to by positive experiences beyond childhood.

By way of contrast, Kernberg (1977) writes about the narcissistic patient's reaction to the past:

> In short, the narcissistic patient has no gratitude for what he has re-
> ceived in the past, experiences the past as lost, wishes he had it now, and is
> painfully resentful that it is no longer available to him. At the bottom, the
> narcissistic patient is painfully envious of himself in the past, having had
> what he no longer has now. (p. 9)

A hallmark of the mature, authentic self is the ability to appraise the personal past with a minimum of denial and distortion. For example, one patient in his forties recognized with clarity for the first time that he grew up in a relatively poor area with limited cultural advantages. This recognition was hidden because it caused narcissistic injury to the childhood self. But from the vantage point of midlife, this aspect of his past was a relatively unimportant observation which could be more easily accepted.

Life in the *present* strongly influences attitudes toward the past and future. Midlife is that phase in which a long sequence of development and maturation has either produced considerable internal integrity and external achievement—both bringing narcissistic gratification; or fragmentation and frustration—bringing pain. There is a strong sense of the present in midlife, an urgency to live life fully *now*.

If the present is sufficiently gratifying, one is more likely to experience nostalgia about the past; if not, envy of the past, as Kernberg describes. For the healthy person the past may be viewed as follows: "Yes, I could have done it differently, even better; but things are pretty good now." The narcissistic sting (envy) is minimized.

There is a normative urge to retain aspects of the youthful self well into midlife. The 50-year old says, "I *feel* the same as I always did." This is both a denial of the aging process and a reflection of the integrity of the adult self resulting from the lifelong process of separation-individuation and the continual reworking of narcissistic issues.

The *future* is also viewed in a new way and gains a special connection with the present and the past through the experience of *continuity*. Relationships and activities that have existed over a period of time connect the personal past with the present and future. Continuity becomes an organizing factor by connecting memories from different ages.

In the normal situation the authentic sense of the past and present allows the healthy individual to view the *future* with a sense of anticipation and minimal amount of fear, for it holds the prospect of even greater gratification as well as the inevitable end of all gratification through death. Among the anticipated pleasures are genuine intimacy, increased wisdom and understanding, and continued involvement in the world in new and productive ways.

Creativity, Mentorship, and Authenticity

Work, which has only been studied superficially, is a central, definitive activity of adulthood and an important component of the self. To illustrate the effect of work on the development of the self, we have chosen to focus on creativity and on mentor relationships. As described in Chapter 4 mentors are those from whom young adults develop *new* aspects of identity. For many individuals, a close relationship with a mentor is a crucial factor in the choice of a career, be it scientist, housewife, waiter, factory worker, or therapist. Although in part based on infantile identifications, this adult process is not a replication of the parent-child relationship. Although early identifications help build psychic structure, later identifications such as the mentor relationship add *specificity* to the adult personality, in this instance through the establishment of a work identity. The process seems to involve three phases: (1) an initial fusion with the mentor, (2) a middle phase in which, through partial identifications, aspects of the mentor are internalized within the self, and finally (3) a separation leading to further individuation.

As far as we know, the role of narcissistic issues in mentor relationships has not been described. In the initial phase the mentor is idealized, as the internal representation of the mentor is invested with narcissism displaced from the self. The sense of fusion during the middle phase brings great pleasure but leaves the self vulnerable since the mentor's approval is necessary for a sense of well-being. The self is dramatically changed as the desired attributes of the mentor are incorporated, usually with intense pleasure. During the separation process considerable pain is experienced, but after a period of working through, the self emerges stronger, enhanced by the greater sense of individuation and capability.

Becoming a mentor is an important task of midlife which involves the painful realization of eventual replacement by another, likely a student. Aggression toward the usurper must be sublimated into a facilitating, teaching role. Conflictual feelings extend not only to the younger person but to his work as well. The capacity to facilitate what is new and valuable independent of its creator must be developed. In the maturing person, particularly the mentor, this process does not occur easily because of the wish to devalue that which was not created by the self, particularly when time or other limitations reduce the capacity of the self to create.

The Return of the Grandiose Self

In response to the basic issues of midlife discussed in this paper, we hypothesize a *reemergence of aspects of infantile narcissism*, which we will describe by utilizing Kohut's concept of the grandiose self. Kohut (1971) originated this concept in his attempt to understand very disturbed patients. It refers to the archaic inflated self-configurations and archaic, overestimated representations of others which have not been integrated into the personality. The result is an impoverishment of the adult personality and its mature functions because of the deprivation of energies which are invested in the ancient structures and a hampering of adult, realistic activities because of the breakthrough and intrusion of archaic representations and claims. A similar (but not the same) process occurs normatively, we believe, in well-integrated individuals in a futile but understandable search for reunion with the omnipotent mother of the first few years who magically controls all aspects of life.

We observe four steps in this process:

Step 1: The return of the aspects of the grandiose self as a narcissistic defense against the aging process, including the growing awareness of time limitation and personal death.

Step 2: A conflict between the regressive wish to accept the return of the grandiose self and the mature urges to reject or reintegrate it within the adult self.

Step 3: Mourning for the loss of the narcissistic gratification promised by the return of the grandiose self.

Step 4: Alteration of the adult self with enhanced individuation and identity formation.

There are a number of possible responses to this increase in infantile narcissism. Some individuals react to the realization of impermanence by trying to increase their control over current life situations. Although accompanied by increased reflectiveness and a clearer appraisal of the relationship between the self and the environment, the need to maintain the status quo may stifle creativity and positive change. In others the conflict may stimulate growth and creativity. The tempering of infantile grandiosity causes a reappraisal of the value of relationships and the importance of current activities, and may lead to major reorganizations in marriage and friendships as well as career and living environment.

When grandiose tendencies are pronounced, the conflict may result in pathological activity such as stagnation, regression, and self-limitation. Persons of either sex may abandon adult responsibilities and long-standing relationships. This behavior is in conflict with the awareness on the part of the authentic self of its interdependence with significant objects such as family, parents, friends, and colleagues. The very depth of these ties may precipitate the inappropriate flight since the self cannot avoid the growing awareness of the passage of time demonstrated by changes such as the death of parents, aging of spouse and friends, and the maturation and growth of children. The ability to remain invested in important loved ones in the face of the narcissistic injury involved in their change is a central developmental task of midlife.

> A woman in the midst of a midlife crisis that was precipitated by the possibility of a malignancy and sterilization expressed a strong desire to have an open marriage, that is, free and ready accessibility to multiple sexual partners before it was too late. "I don't think I'm going to live past 45." She wished to move into a small apartment separate from her husband and children. There, in splendid isolation, her needs would be paramount. For example, she imagined sitting alone in restaurants, having the exclusive attention of waiters.

In this woman the potential threat to her sexuality and increased fear of dying caused the strong emergence of wishes to be an infant, protected and gratified by an all-giving mother. However, another set of factors also played a part: she expressed fears of turning into the angry, "bitchy" menopausal mother of her adolescence, "the old woman." In this fear, the patient clearly illustrates Greenson's (1950) useful clinical concept of a struggle against identification since, in response to aging, she felt she was becoming the parent of her adolescence. The defense against becoming like "that bitchy menopausal woman" was to have affairs in a symbolic attempt to deny the aging process. This patient not only illustrates a regressive response to the return of the grandiose self but a failure to integrate adult oedipal phenomena. A full understanding of the relationship between these adult themes and the genetic antecedents of childhood provided the patient

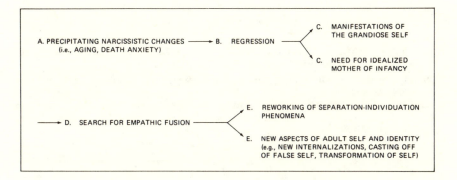

FIGURE 4. Midlife model of reworking of adult self.

and therapist with meaningful insight. In Figure 4 we have constructed a schematic model of those midlife processes.

SUMMARY

In this chapter we have defined characteristics of the self in adulthood and described the factors that shape it, focusing particularly on the role of narcissism in the shaping process. The concepts we have presented are based on the hypothesis that the self in adulthood is not a static, finished product but is in a state of dynamic flux and change within the developmental continuum.

We chose the term "authentic" to characterize the mature adult self because it describes the capacity to accept what is genuine within the self and the outer world regardless of the narcissistic injury involved. The capacity for authenticity emerges out of the developmental experiences of childhood and adulthood. Among the most important influences in adulthood are narcissistic issues related to (1) the aging body, (2) significant relationships, particularly with spouse, children, and parents, (3) middle-age time sense, and (4) the vicissitudes of work and creativity.

We conceptualized a normal narcissistic regression precipitated by the confrontation with these developmental tasks of midlife leading to a reemergence of aspects of infantile narcissism, which we characterized by using Kohut's concept of the grandiose self. The reworking and eventual integration of aspects of the infantile grandiosity are seen by us as an integral part of normal development in midlife.

REFERENCES

Benedek, T., & Maranon, G. The climacteric. In A. M. Karch (Ed.), *Men: The variety and meaning of the sexual experience.* New York: Dell, 1954.

Blos, P. The second individuation process of adolescence. *Psychoanalytic Study of the Child,* 1967, *22*, 162.

Cath, S. H. Grief, loss and emotional disorders in the aging process. In M. A. Berezin & S. H. Cath (Eds.), *Geriatric psychiatry.* New York: International Universities Press, 1962, pp. 21–72.

Colarusso, C. A., & Nemiroff, R. A. Some observations and hypotheses about the psychoanalytic theory of adult development. *International Journal of Psycho-Analysis,* 1979, *60,* 59.

Eissler, K. On possible effects of aging on the practice of psychoanalysis: An essay. *Journal of the Philadelphia Association for Psychoanalysis,* 1975, *11,* 139.

Erikson, E. H. Eight ages of man. In *Childhood and society.* New York: W. W. Norton, 1963, pp. 247–269.

Freud, S. *Instincts and their vicissitudes.* Standard edition 14:109. London: Hogarth Press, 1915.

Greenson, R. R. The struggle against identification. *Journal of the American Psychoanalytic Association,* 1950, *2,* 200.

Jacobson, E. *The self and the object world.* New York: International Universities Press, 1965.

Jacques, E. Death and the mid-life crisis. *International Journal of Psycho-Analysis,* 1965, *46,* 602.

Kernberg, O. *Pathological narcissism in middle age.* Paper presented at annual meeting of the American Psychoanalytic Association, May 1977, Quebec.

Kohut, H. *The analysis of the self.* New York: International Universities Press, 1971.

Kramer, P. On discovering one's identity: A case report. *Psychoanalytic Study of the Child,* 1955, *10,* 47.

Lichtenberg, J. D. The development of the sense of self. *Journal of the American Psychoanalytic Association,* 1975, *23,* 453.

Lichtenstein, H. Identity and sexuality, a study of their inter-relationships. *Journal of the American Psychoanalytic Association,* 1961, *9,* 179.

Loewald, H. On the nature of the therapeutic action of psychoanalysis. *International Journal of Psycho-Analysis,* 1960, *41,* 54.

Mahler, M. In M. Winestine (Reporter), The experience of separation-individuation . . . through the course of life: Infancy and childhood (Panel report). *Journal of the American Psychoanalytic Association,* 1973, *21,* 135.

Marcus, J. (Reporter). The experience of separation-individuation . . . through the course of life: Adolescence and maturity (Panel report). *Journal of the American Psychoanalytic Association,* 1973, *21,* 155.

Moore, B., & Fine, B. *A glossary of psychoanalytic terms and concepts.* New York: American Psychoanalytic Association, 1968.

Pollock, G. H. Mourning and adaptation. *International Journal of Psycho-Analysis,* 1961, *42,* 341.

Pribram, K. Neural modifiability and memory mechanisms. In *Languages of the brain: Experimental paradoxes and principles in neuropsychology.* Englewood Cliffs, N.J.: Prentice-Hall, 1971, pp. 3–47.

Rosenblatt, A., & Thickstun, J. *Modern psychoanalytic concepts in a general psychology.* New York: International Universities Press, 1977.

Saperstein, J. L., & Gaines, J. Metapsychological considerations of the self. *International Journal of Psycho-Analysis*, 1973, 54, 415.

Shafer, R. Concepts of self and identity, and of separation-individuation in adolescence. *Psychoanalytic Quarterly*, 1973, 42, 42.

Steinschein, I. (Reporter). The experience of separation-individuation . . . through the course of life: Maturity, senescence, and sociological implications (Panel report). *Journal of the American Psychoanalytic Association*, 1973, 21, 633.

Sutherland, J. *The self and personal object relations.* Unpublished manuscript, 1978.

Winestine, M. (Reporter). The experience of separation-individuation . . . through the course of life: Infancy and childhood (Panel report). *Journal of the American Psychoanalytic Association*, 1973, 21, 135.

6

Myths about the Aging Body

In Chapter 4 we asked the question, "What are the normal biological and maturational events of adulthood, and how would awareness of them help us achieve a more complete understanding of mental development?" After discussing the prevailing attitude that a detailed knowledge of biological processes would not contribute to an expanded dynamic theory of adulthood, we presented some research on the adult brain, primarily by Pribram (1971), which indicated that current ideas on the functioning of the brain might be very limited.

Since writing the paper that was the basis for that chapter, we have completed a comprehensive computer survey of the available literature on the *normal* functioning of the adult body and brain. The findings have resulted in our calling this chapter "Myths about the Aging Body," since so many of the basic tenets that underlie popular concepts about the brain—and mental functioning—are being questioned. In this chapter we plan to present a summary of the most recent studies available on the functioning of the adult body and brain to provide a data bank for ourselves and others from which to elaborate a psychodynamic theory of mind–body interaction in adulthood.

SEXUAL MYTHS

Myth: The Menopausal Syndrome Is Caused by Estrogen Deficiency

The upsurge of sexual hormones at puberty leads to profound biological change which is followed by equally significant psychological

This chapter was written with David R. Talley, M.D., who was a senior medical student at the University of California at San Diego at the time.

change—the period of development we call adolescence. At no point in the life cycle is a causal relationship between biological events and psychological response clearer. At first glance it appears that a similar situation, but in reverse, exists at the time of the climacteric when the *loss* of sexual hormones produces in women a major psychobiological response called "the menopausal syndrome." However, current research indicates that the similarity between adolescence and the climacteric is superficial at best. In adulthood the relationship between loss of sexual hormones and personality change is unclear, particularly in regard to a simple cause-and-effect relationship between estrogen deficiency and the menopausal syndrome.

The female climacteric usually occurs in the fifth or sixth decade. The menopause, or cessation of menses, is the external manifestation of a gradual decrease in hormone production. A study of premenopausal women who are still having regular menstrual cycles (Sherman, West, & Korman, 1976) showed decreased levels of estradiol (E_2) concentration, increased levels of follicle-stimulating hormone (FSH), and normal levels of luteinizing hormone (LH). The onset of the menopause is evidenced by a much greater decrease in E_2, a decrease in progesterone, and further increases in LH and FSH. When a woman becomes postmenopausal she continues to produce some estrogen through the peripheral conversion of adrenal androsteinedione; but her total estrogen levels are much lower than those of her premenopausal sisters. The diminished hormone production applies to androgens as well since the aging female also has significantly decreased levels of adrenal androgens (dehydroepiandrosterone and androsterone)(Gregerman & Bierman, 1974).

This dramatic decrease in estrogens occurring during the climacteric has long been associated in the minds of physicians and the lay public with a set of physical and emotional symptoms—the menopausal syndrome—which include hot flashes, depression, anxiety, irritability, emotional lability, insomnia, and increased somatic complaints. However, the endocrinological basis, indeed the very existence of a menopausal syndrome, has been challenged. The assumption that the syndrome was caused by estrogen deficiency was first attacked 40 years ago by Pratt and Thomas (1937), who showed that relief of the behavioral-emotional symptoms associated with the menopause occurred *equally* with estrogen, barbiturates, and placebos. More recently, Neugarten and Kraines (1965), after completing a comprehensive, cross-generational study, came to similar conclusions. Referring to that and other studies, Eisdorfer and Raskind (1975), who surveyed the literature, report:

> Menopausal women (age 45 to 54) noted a higher incidence of somatic complaints, whereas adolescents (age 14 to 19) reported higher incidence of psychological complaints. Specific symptoms noted more frequently by the menopausal group included hot flashes, paresthesias and palpitations. Surprisingly, the common "menopausal" symptoms, such as irritability, nervousness, depression, insomnia and crying spells, were reported with a frequency *equal to or lower* by the menopausal group than by the other groups examined. The postmenopausal group (age 55 to 64), presumably with the lowest estrogen production levels, reported the lowest incidence of tired feelings, headaches, dizzy spells, irritability and nervousness, depression, crying spells and difficulty concentrating. (p. 380, italics added)

These studies suggest that the menopausal syndrome, if it does exist, cannot be attributed to estrogen depletion, except for those symptoms with a clear somatic basis, that is, the hot flashes of vasomotor instability. It is our hypothesis that most menopausal symptoms may be psychologically based, occurring in those women with an exaggerated response to phase-specific developmental events such as loss of fertility, aging of the body, and loss of the mothering function. The implications for treatment are significant. Diagnosis and treatment should be based on a combined psychobiological approach which assumes that the reasons for the occurrence of the symptoms are more complex than simple hormone loss and that treatment must do more than replace the hormone loss. A combination of dynamic psychotherapy and hormone replacement is probably indicated in most cases.

Myth: Postmenopausal Women Cannot Enjoy Sex because of the Physiological and Psychological Effects of Estrogen Withdrawal

In the minds of many, elderly women gradually become asexual, primarily because of the physical and psychological changes produced by diminished estrogen production. A direct relationship is assumed between aging and loss of sexual interest and ability.

Understanding of the physiological changes that occur with age in the normal, healthy woman was greatly increased by the important work of Masters and Johnson, *Human Sexual Response* (1966). Their research showed definite changes in the sexual organs of older women attributable to diminished estrogen production. These included thinning of the vaginal mucosa and a decrease in the rate and amount of lubrication production. Other changes discovered were decreases in vaginal length, width, and elasticity and a small decrease in the number of contractions with orgasm. Some women reported dyspareunia and dysuria resulting from thinning of the vaginal mucosa, diminished lubrication and decreased distensibility of the vaginal barrel, while a few developed painful uterine contractions during and after orgasm, all of which were relieved by estrogen and progesterone replacement. But these changes were not universally present. Three elderly women, in their sixties and seventies, possessed the same lubricating abilities as women in their twenties and were not subject to the complaints of their peers. Significantly, they were the *only* women in the over 60 age group who had maintained regular sexual activity at least weekly throughout their adult years.

The conclusion is obvious. Estrogen depletion is only one factor, and a reversible one at that, determining the sexual capacity of the elderly woman. Her *attitude* toward sexuality (which is determined in part by what is expected and allowed by society) and the *availability* of a sexual partner are the most important factors determining the presence or absence of a gratifying sexual life.

To quote Masters and Johnson (1966):

> Thus the simple fact remains that if opportunity for regularity of coital exposure is created or maintained, the elderly woman suffering from all of the vaginal stigmas of sex-steroid starvation still will retain a far higher capacity for sexual performance than her female counterpart who does not have similar coital opportunities. (pp. 241–242)

It is clear that the therapist who treats the elderly woman as a dried-up, asexual "prune" will be perpetrating a long-standing, harmful myth and may be doing his patient a disservice by ignoring such vital factors as sexual attitudes, physical health, and the availability of sexual partners.

Myth: A Decrease in Testosterone Levels is Responsible for the Decline in Sexual Functioning in Older Men

To the present, research has not established clearly delineated, widely accepted normal levels of sexual hormones in adult men. Estrogen levels, for example, have been described as decreasing (Gregerman & Bierman, 1974), increasing (Harman, 1978), and remaining the same

(Mandell, 1979) with aging. The results are just as varied for testosterone levels. In 1972, Vermeulen, Rubens, and Verdonck reported a progressive decline in mean serum-testosterone levels after the age of 50. However, there was marked variation within age groups. Some men in the 80–90 age group had levels as low as women, whereas the levels in others equaled the mean in the 20–30 age group. A very recently reported longitudinal study by Harman (1979) conducted on men of ages 25 to 89 found *no* decrease in testosterone or free-testosterone levels after the age of 30. (Increases in LH, FSH, and FSH/LH were noted, however.) Harman offered an explanation for the discrepancy between his study and earlier ones: "Most of the earlier studies recruited old men from clinics of hospitals, men whose disorders may have influenced androgen levels". In contrast, his subjects were "healthy, active men who were neither alcoholic nor obese" (p. 11). If Harman's results are duplicated by other research, a major shift will be required in our thinking about sexual functioning and attitudes in healthy older men. The importance of good health as a major determinant of development in middle and late adulthood is becoming increasingly clear, as is the debilitating effect of illness.

The relationship between testosterone levels and sexual functioning and aggression is just as unclear as the relationship between testosterone levels and aging. Consider the following contradictory studies. Sachar, Halpern, Rosenfelt, Gallagher, and Hellman (1973) found no correlation among testosterone levels, libido, and aggressiveness in depressed men. On the other hand, Persky, Smith, and Basu (1971) reported that testosterone production was correlated with aggression in young men (mean age 22 years) but not in older men (mean age 45 years). A positive correlation between high levels of free testosterone and increased sexual activity in all age groups was found by Harman (1979), but a simple cause-and-effect relationship may not be involved. A study of testosterone levels in a 38-year-old man (Fox, Ismail, Love, Kirkham, & Loraine, 1972) revealed increases during and after intercourse, suggesting that the elevated testosterone levels were a result of sexual activity rather than a cause of it.

The lack of clear-cut evidence of a decrease in testosterone production with age, and uncertainty about the relationship between testosterone levels and sexual functioning, cast doubt upon a simple biological etiology for the decline in male sexual function with age. In addition, it appears that there is no male analogy to the female climacteric with its dramatic decrease in sex steroids over a relatively short period of time. The so-called male menopause, a condition that supposedly afflicts men in their forties and fifties with nervousness, irritability, decreased memory and concentration, somatic complaints, depression, decreased sexual potency, loss of self-confidence, and an increased likelihood of extramarital affairs, usually with much younger women (Sheehy, 1974), most certainly is not caused by significant changes in plasma-testosterone levels. The relationship between testosterone levels and sexual function is essentially unknown. Even when this information becomes available, the relationship between hormones and sexual functioning will not be fully understood because there is a gradual increase in impotence after age 35, affecting 50% of men by age 75.

It is open to question, however, whether this increase in secondary impotence is primarily physiological or functional. A study (Karacan, Williams, Thornby, & Salis, 1975) of sleep-related erections in males aged three to 79 found a peak in the second decade, a rapid decrease in the third and fourth decades, and only a gradual decrease thereafter through the eighth decade. This study suggests a largely functional etiology. As noted by Masters and Johnson (1966):

> The fear of performance reflecting cultural stigmas directed toward erective inadequacy was that associated with problems of secondary impotence. These fears were expressed, under interrogation, by every male study subject beyond forty years of age, irrespective of reported levels of formal education. Regardless of whether the individual male study subject had ever experienced an instance of erective difficulty, the probability that secondary impotence was associated directly with the aging process was vocalized constantly. The fallacy that secondary impotence is to be expected as the male ages is probably more firmly entrenched in our culture than any other misapprehension . . . . In most instances, secondary impotence is a reversible process for all men regardless of age, unless there is a background of specific injury or physical trauma. (pp. 203–204)

MYTHS ABOUT THE BRAIN AND MENTAL FUNCTION

Myth: Intelligence Reaches a Peak in the Twenties and Then Declines at a Steady Rate

The issue of changes in intelligence with age is very controversial, in part because of a lack of agreement among investigators as to exactly what comprises "intelligence." Eisdorfer (1978) provides a survey of the research in this area for the reader who wishes more information than is presented here. Wechsler (1941) described a pattern of decreasing intellectual ability with age:

> the data show that intellectual ability after reaching a maximum at 20–25 does not continue unaltered for any length of time but starts trailing off immediately thereafter. Beginning at age 30, the rate of decline maintains almost a constant slope. Intellectual decline follows the same general decline as does physical ability. (p. 46)

Wechsler's cross-sectional study has been disproven by longitudinal studies of intelligence which now extend over a 40-year period. The essence of this research is simple and is contained in the following quotation from Jarvik (1973): "if illness does not intervene, cognitive stability is the rule and can be maintained into the ninth decade" (p. 67). Eisdorfer (1978) sums up the current status of the controversy:

> There are now data from a number of studies which question [Wechsler's] conclusions (Bates and Schail, 1974; Bayley and Oden, 1955; Rhudnick and Gordon, 1973) and which have produced evidence that there is no clear peaking of intelligence with age during the third decade of life.

Even Botwinick (1977) and Horn (1975), who have been major proponents of the hypothesis supporting the decline of intelligence in adulthood, agree that there is no simple unidimensional drop in intelligence past the third decade of life. The question, then, as stated by Eisdorfer, becomes "not so much decline versus no decline, but a matter of what, if any, components decline, and when and under what conditions, if at all, decline is observed" (p. 110).

This startling reversal of attitude, which indicates that, *in the presence of good health,* middle and old age can be times of intellectual stability and growth, has wide implications in general and for the mental-health profession in particular. It underscores the importance of (1) preventive medicine to ensure good physical health, and (2) the maintenance of a level of mental activity and interpersonal involvement in peoples of all ages. Additionally, the growth of intellectual capacity with age and experience should change the basic attitude of the therapist toward his older patients from one of supportive maintenance to one of dynamic respect for a patient who is capable of intellectual curiosity about himself and the world.

As the following section demonstrates, the idea of *decline with aging* permeates scientific and lay thinking about brain functioning just as it does for mental and sexual functioning.

Myth: The Aging Brain Loses Weight and Neurons and Demonstrates Inevitable Senile Changes

Ordy and Schjeide (1973) summarize the morphological changes seen in the brain with aging. They report a cumulative loss of approximately 50,000 neurons per day (cumulative because neurons are incapable of reproduction) and structural changes in the remaining neurons.

> These include changes in size, nuclear-cytoplasmic ratios, accumulation of lipofuscia pigment, decreases in Nissl substance (rough endoplasmic reticulum), mitochondria, mirotubules, neurofilaments, and ribonuclear proteins. (p. 31)

In addition,

> In man, there is also a 10% reduction from 1300 to 1170 grams in brain weight from 60 to 80 years of age, an increase in the size of the ventricles, calcification in the meninges, and reduction in the sulci and gyri of the cerebral hemispheres. (p. 31)

The picture is clearly one of cellular loss and degeneration.

Many of the studies in our survey of the literature which express the prevalent ideas and attitudes about the aging brain have recently been challenged.

Dayan (1972) has made a survey of the recent evidence on the question of neuronal loss with aging. It is his conclusion that "earlier evidence suggesting fallout of neurones [sic] has been disproven at almost every major anatomical site where exact counts have been made" (p. 64). For example, Konigsmark and Murphy (1972) did careful cell counts in the ventral cochlear nuclei of 23 brains from neurologically normal subjects ranging in age from newborn to 90 years. They found *no* decrease in neurons with age. These researchers criticized Brody's (1955) conclusion that brain loses 50,000 neurons per day on the grounds that it was based on a very small number of cases and a sampling of only 0.005% of the cerebral cortex.

An inevitable decline in brain weight with age has also been questioned. Tomlinson (1972), in a study of 28 intellectually well-preserved individuals aged 65 to 92, found no significant decrease in brain weight with age. He stated that earlier studies with contradictory findings sampled an atypical population base since they often used brains from mental-institution patients. Howard (1973) made the point that the decrease in brain weight with aging may be artifactual change caused by chronic disease rather than age. She cited studies (Appel & Appel,

1942, Blakerman, 1905) showing that *cause of death* is better correlated with brain weight than is age.

Tomlinson (1972) also studied the incidence of senile changes in his population of elderly brains, mean age 75 years. Cortical atrophy was present in 54%, but only 14% showed more than slight changes. Forty percent showed enlargement of the ventricles, while 39% had either no plaques or an extremely small number. Forty-six percent were essentially free of neurofibrillary tangles. In those brains with plaques and/or neurofibrillary tangles, the majority of the changes were restricted to the hippocampus. Thus even in an aged population, senile changes are by no means inevitable. It is also of interest that the majority of the changes were confined to the hippocampus, a portion of the brain thought to be involved in the consolidation of memory—especially in light of the decline in short-term memory seen with aging.

It is clear from the research that a global decline in brain structure is not a necessary consequence of aging. Instead the possibility has been raised that there is remarkably little change in brain morphology with age and that when degenerative change is present it may be attributable to illness or marked inactivity (as in mental patients) rather than to aging. Again the point is made, this time on the level of brain functioning, that advanced age itself is not synonymous with central-nervous-system decline or diminished mental capacity. Older patients must be individually assessed to determine their capacities for mental and emotional functioning.

Myth: The Adult Brain is a Finished Product, Incapable of Structural Change

Just as the adult personality is considered to be static and unchanging, so is the adult brain. This basic attitude toward the adult personality and brain has, we feel, impeded the study of these areas and the *interconnections* between them. It is obvious that we seriously question the belief that the adult personality is rigid and finished. Evidence is now appearing about the adult brain which is just as dramatic and dynamic, for recent work has raised the possibility of change in brain structure in response to stimulation, that is, experiences in living. The concept of *neural plasticity* is the key to understanding this possibility.

One particular form of plasticity involves the formation of new synapses in adult brains, a "rewiring" of the brain. All current evidence is from studies on laboratory animals; the invasive nature of the work makes it impossible to use human subjects. This fact does raise important, as yet unanswerable, questions about the applicability of the findings to humans.

Bennett and colleagues (Bennett & Rosenweig, 1970; Bennett, Diamond, Krech, & Rosenweig, 1964) discovered that rats reared in a high-stimulation environment showed a significant thickening of the cortex when compared to rats raised in a more restrictive environment. Microscopically, the more stimulated rats had increased numbers of glial cells, dendritic spines, and branching of basal dendrites. The dendritic changes would seem to indicate synaptic modification in response to stimulation. Other studies have shown that the capacity to respond to increased environmental stimulation is retained in adult rats, although it is somewhat attenuated (Bennett & Rosenweig, 1970; Latorre, 1968).

Another form of neural plasticity defined by Lund (1978) involves the peripheral nervous system, where damage to a nerve is likely to result in sprouting of adjacent, intact nerves that invade the denervated area. This phenomenon is termed *collateral sprouting*. A study by Cotman and Scheff (1979) examined sprouting in CNS neurons in both young and old rats. Lesions were made in the entorhinal area of the brain, whence efferent nerve fibers project to a well-described region of the hippocampal dentate gyrus. The death of the entorhinal neurons results in a precipitous loss of synapses in the hippocampal dentate gyrus. However, after approximately 240 days the number of synapses had returned to normal. Upon electromicrographic study the affected area of the dentate gyrus looked almost normal, with only slight distortion of the dendrites. Further examination, however, showed that only a few of the new synapses were made up of fibers from the contralateral entorhinal cortex; the rest were from nearby commissural areas and other associational fibers. Thus, a whole new pattern of input was created. The new synapses appeared to be functional on electrophysiological studies. Surprisingly, the new, functional afferent fibers had different neurotransmitters—ACH and aspartate instead of glutamate. In aged rats, the course of events was similar, except for a slower rate of recovery, a decrease in the number of synapses, and differences in appearance of the new synapses. Again, there was decreased capacity but not loss of plasticity with age.

Sprouting offers a potential mechanism whereby the "wiring" of the adult brain can change in spite of the lack of reproductive ability in the neurons. However, Lund (1978) qualifies these findings for the human brain. "The question of *de novo* synapse formation in adult brains remains to be shown and its presence to be demonstrated before one can safely expect synaptic mobility to play a significant role in memory and behavior" (pp. 302–303).

Lund's careful qualification tells us that we do not have enough evidence to assume that synaptic mobility occurs in man or that it plays a significant part in mental functioning and behavior. This is a question for the future. But the work referred to here does raise the distinct possibility that our current concept of the adult brain as static and slowly degenerating may be as dated as the idea that the earth is flat.

Summary

American society associates old age with a dramatic decrease in sexual interest and activity. A 1975 Harris poll sponsored by the National Council on Aging revealed that although 74% of the public felt that people over 65 were "warm and friendly" and 64% viewed them as "wise from experience," only 5% considered them "very sexually active." Interestingly, those over 65 tend to view themselves as more sexually active than do those who are younger. This widely held view of greatly diminished sexuality in old age is not biologically mandated, but is nevertheless a disturbingly accurate assessment of the current sexual behavior of the elderly.

Harman (1978) surveyed the literature on changes in sexual behavior with aging. He referred to a study by Martin (1977) involving well-educated, white, middle-class males which showed a steady decrease in the frequency of orgasms (coital and masturbatory) with age, from a peak of 600 sexual events per five-year period for men aged 30 to 34, to 100 sexual events per five-year period for the 75- to 79-year-old age group. Citing a number of other studies, Harman also found a corresponding decrease in sexual activity in women. In both sexes there was a close correlation between present and past levels of sexual activity. The most important factor in determining the level of sexual activity with age appears to be the health and survival of the spouse, and the second most important factor is the health of the subject himself. Although sexual interest tends to decrease with age, it always remains significantly greater than activity—a fact that manages to be both reassuring and somewhat disappointing.

Some degree of declining sexual function and interest appears to be an inevitable consequence of aging, but health, social, and cultural factors rather than the physiological changes of aging per se seem to be responsible for most of the sexual changes seen with aging. It is difficult to separate the purely biological factors from the psychosocial ones, but it does seem clear that satisfying sexual activity is possible for reasonably healthy people regardless of age. Sad to say, for the majority of the elderly this potential is not realized. The widely held view that the elderly are essentially asexual, although it is biologically unsound, is at this time more or less a self-fulfilling prophecy.

Prevalent attitudes about the functioning of the brain in middle and late adulthood seem just as skewed as those about sexual functioning. Recent research indicates that mental functioning need not necessarily decline with age because of inevitable degenerative changes in the brain. Physical health and social factors such as the availability of interpersonal relationships and environmental stimulation determine the course of mental development in middle and late adulthood rather than inevitable central-nervous-system decline.

The challenges for students of human behavior rising from these ideas are multiple and exciting. Therapists must shed misconceptions about middle- and late-adulthood patients and develop a new respect for their mental and sexual capabilities and potential for dynamic, explorative psychotherapy.

But the most exciting challenge lies in the integration of the newly emerging ideas on body functioning with those on mental functioning. In Chapter 4 we noted the absence of a defined theory of mind—body interaction for adulthood and questioned statements by Freud (1915) and Rapaport (1960) that knowledge of somatic processes is unnecesary for the elaboration of a theory of mental functioning. In our opinion the integration of biological research on the normal functioning of the body and brain with dynamic theories of mental functioning, leading to the elaboration of an integrated theory of mind–body interaction for the entire life cycle, is one of the most exciting challenges facing students of human behavior.

References

Appel, F. W., & Appel, E. M. Intracranial variation in the weight of the human brain. *Human Biology,* 1942, *14,* 235.

Bates, P. B., & Schail, K. W. Aging and IQ: The myth of the twilight years. *Psychology Today,* 1974, *7,* 35.

Bayley, N., & Oden, M. H. The maintenance of intellectual ability in gifted adults. *Journal of Gerontology,* 1955, *10,* 91.

Bennett, E. L., & Rosenweig, M. R. Chemical alterations produced in brain by environment and training. In A. Lajtha (Ed.), *Handbook of neurochemistry.* New York: Plenum Press, 1970.

Bennett, E. L., Diamond, M. C., Krech, D., & Rosenweig, M. R. Chemical and anatomical plasticity of the brain. *Science,* 1964, *146,* 610.

Blakerman, J. A study of the biometric constants of English brain-weights, and their relationships to external physical measurements. *Biometrika,* 1905, *4,* 124.

Botwinick, J. Intellectual abilities. In J. E. Birren & K. W. Schail (Eds.), *Handbook of the psychology of aging.* New York: Van Nostrand Reinhold, 1977, pp. 580–602.

Brody, H. Organization of the cerebral cortex, Ill. A study of aging in the human cortex. *Journal of Comparative Neurology,* 1955, *102,* 511.

Cotman, C. W., & Scheff, S. W. Synaptic growth in aged animals. In A. Cherkin (Eds.), *Physiology and cell biology of aging* (Vol. 8). New York: Raven Press, 1979, pp. 109–120.

Dayan, A. D. The brain and theories of aging. In A. M. Van Praag & A. F. Kalverboer (Eds.), *Aging and the central nervous system: Biological and psychological aspects.* Haarlem, The Netherlands: DeErvan F. Bohn N.V., 1972, pp. 58–75.

Eisdorfer, C. Psychophysiologic and cognitive studies in the aged. In G. Usdin & C. S. Hofling (Eds.), *Aging: The process and the people.* New York: Brunner/Mazel, 1978, pp. 96–128.

Eisdorfer, C., & Raskind, R. Aging and human behavior. In B. E. Eleftreriois & R. L. Spratt (Eds.), *Hormonal correlates of behavior,* Vol. 1. *A lifespan view.* New York: Plenum Press, 1975, pp. 369–387.

Fox, C. A., Ismail, A. A. A., Love, D. N., Kirkham, K. E., & Loraine, J. A. Studies on the relationship between plasma testosterone levels and human sexual activity. *Journal of Endocrinology,* 1972, *52,* 51.

Freud, S. *Instincts and their vicissitudes,* Standard edition, 14:109. London: Hogarth Press, 1915.

Gregerman, R. I., & Bierman, E. L. Aging and hormones. In R. H. Williams (Ed.), *Textbook of endocrinology.* Philadelphia: W. B. Saunders, 1974, pp. 1059–1069.

Harman, S. M. Clinical aspects of aging of the male reproductive system. In E. L. Schneider (Ed.), *Aging,* Vol. 4. *The aging reproductive system.* New York: Raven Press, 1978, pp. 29–58.

Harman, S. W. Male menopause? The hormones flow but sex does slow. *Medical World News,* 1979, *20,* 11.

Horn, J. L. Psychometric studies of aging and intelligence. In S. Gershon & A. Raskin (Eds.), *Genesis and treatment of psychological disorders in the elderly.* New York: Raven Press, 1975, pp. 19–43.

Howard, E. DNA content of rodent brains, during maturation and aging, and autoradiography of postnatal DNA synthesis in monkey brain. In D. H. Ford (Ed.), *Neurobiological aspects of maturation and aging.* New York: Elsevier, 1973, pp. 91–114.

Jarvik, L. F. Intellectual functioning in later years. In L. F. Jarvik, C. Eisdorfer, & J. E. E. Blum (Eds.), *Intellectual functioning in adults.* New York: Springer, 1973, p. 67.

Karacan, I., Williams R. L., Thornby, J. I., & Salis, P. J. Sleep-related penile tumescence as a function of age. *American Journal of Psychiatry*, 1975, *132*, 932.

Kinsey, A. C., Pomeroy, W. B., & Martin, C. E. *Sexual behavior in the human male*. Philadelphia: W. B. Saunders, 1948, p. 23.

Konigsmark, B. W., & Murphy, E. A. Volume of the ventral cochlear nucleus in man: Its relationship to neuronal populations and age. *Journal of Neuropathology and Experimental Neurology*, 1972, *31*, 304.

Latorre, J. C. Effect of differential environment enrichment on brain weight and on acetylcholinesterase and cholinesterase activities in mice. *Experimental Neurology*, 1968, *22*, 493.

Lund, R. E. *Development and plasticity of the brain*. New York: Oxford University Press, 1978.

Mandell, A. J. On a mechanism for the mood and personality changes of adult and later life: A psychobiological hypothesis. *Journal of Nervous and Mental Disorders*, 1979, *167*, 457.

Martin, C. E. Sexual activity in the aging male. In J. Money & H. Musaph (Eds.), *Handbook of sexology*. Amsterdam: Elsevier/North-Holland, 1977.

Masters, W., & Johnson, V. *Human sexual response*. London: J. & A. Churchill, 1966, pp. 223–270.

Neugarten, B. L., & Kraines, R. J. Menopausal symptoms in women of various ages. *Psychosomatic Medicine*, 1965, *27*, 266.

Ordy, S. M., & Schjeide, O. A. Univariate and multivariate models for evaluating long term changes in neurobiological development, maturity and aging. In D. H. Ford (Ed.), *Neurological aspects of maturation and aging*. New York: Elsevier, 1973.

Persky, H., Smith, K. D., & Basu, G. K. Relation of psychologic measures of aggression and hostility to testosterone production in man. *Psychosomatic Medicine*, 1971, *33*, 265.

Pratt, J. P., & Thomas, W. L. The endocrine treatment of menopausal phenomena. *Journal of the American Medical Association*, 1937, *109*, 1875.

Pribram, K. Neural modifiability and memory mechanisms. In *Languages of the brain: Experimental paradoxes and principles in neuropsychology*. Englewood Cliffs, N.J.: Prentice-Hall, 1971, pp. 3–47.

Rapaport, D. On the psychoanalytic theory of motivation. In M. R. Jones (Ed.), *Nebraska Symposium on Motivation*. Lincoln: University of Nebraska press, 1960, pp. 173–247.

Rhudnick, P. J., & Gordon, C. The Age Center of New England study. In L. J. Jarvik, C. Eisdorfer, & J. E. Blum (Eds.), *Intellectual functioning in adults*. New York: Springer, 1973, pp. 7–19.

Sachar, E. S., Halpern, F., Rosenfelt, R. S., Gallagher, T. F., & Hellman, L. Plasma and urinary testosterone levels in depressed men. *Archives of General Psychiatry*, 1973, *28*, 15.

Sheehy, G. *Passages*. New York: E. P. Dutton, 1974, pp. 456–462.

Sherman, B. M., West, J. H., & Korenman, S. G. The menopausal transition: Analysis of LH, FHS, estradiol and progesterone concentrations during menstrual cycles of older women. *Journal of Clinical Endocrinology and Metabolism*, 1976, *42*, 629.

Tomlinson, B. E. Morphological brain changes in non-demented old people. In A. M. Van Praag & A. F. Kalverboer (Eds.), *Aging of the central nervous system: Biological and psychological aspects*. Haarlem, The Netherlands: De Erven F. Bohn N.V., 1972, pp. 38–57.

Vermeulen, A., Rubens, R., & Verdonck, L. Testosterone secretion and metabolism in male senescence. *Journal of Clinical Endocrine Metabolism*, 1972, *34*, 730.

Wechsler, D. Intellectual changes with age. *Mental Health in Later Maturity*, Suppl. 168. Federal Security Agency, United States Public Health Service, 1941, pp. 43–52.

7

Male Midlife Crisis

THE GAUGUIN SYNDROME, MYTH AND REALITY

The Gauguin Syndrome

Charles Strickland, the protagonist of Somerset Maugham's novel *The Moon and Sixpence* (1919), which is supposedly based on the life of the painter Paul Gauguin, is one of the great narcissistic villains of literature. As the story goes, Strickland, a successful English banker, suddenly, without warning, abandons his family and his work and goes to Polynesia to be a painter. Like Gauguin, he eventually dies in the tropics. Actually, instead of the classic "Gauguin" scenario of middle-aged man deserting wife, children, and career to escape to the tropics for self-fulfillment and play with exotic, bare-breasted women, we should refer instead to the *myth* of Gauguin since investigation reveals a very different version of the painter's life. The facts suggest a situation of considerable intrapsychic, marital, and occupational complexity. Gauguin was bored with the banking business and felt he had gone as far as he could go. He had been experimenting with a career in art for years, first as a patron of the early impressionists and then as an amateur painter. A considerable period of transition occurred between the two careers. Likewise, his marital problems did not arise suddenly. He and his wife, Mette, had been changing at different rates and in different ways over a span of years—he evolving a mode of self-expression while she became increasingly involved in middle-class society. Before going to Tahiti he spent years imploring her to join him, but she would have none of it.

119

Gauguin's midlife metamorphosis becomes even more under-standable in light of his family background and childhood. His mater-nal grandmother, Flora Tristan, was a fiery revolutionary who eventu-ally came to regard herself as an outcast, a pariah and missionary of social change. There is evidence to suggest that Gauguin *identified* with his grandmother, especially in her revolutionary-outcast role. On his mother's side the family was part of the Peruvian aristocracy; his father died while the family was en route to Peru to join the household of the Peruvian Viceroy, Gauguin's maternal uncle. Part of Gauguin's child-hood was spent in a materially abundant, colorful aristocratic environ-ment in which his mother flourished, and he always retained an image of her in that exotic setting. Later he painted her many times as "Eve" in a tropical paradise. Because of a change in the political situation the Gauguin family abruptly returned to France when Paul was seven. The boy's golden world dissolved, to be replaced by the gray and pallid en-vironment of Orleans. During adolescence Gauguin shipped out as a sailor, as if to try to recapture his early Peruvian experience; while he was at sea his mother died (Anderson, 1971).

Such early experiences, including identification with a grand-mother who was a revolutionary and an outcast, a lifelong yearning for a Peruvian paradise lost, and early separations and deaths likely played some part in his later attempts to master loneliness and separa-tion. Gauguin was thus influenced by powerful emotional forces which seemed to precipitate a midlife attempt to work through his early emo-tional traumata. Mayer (1978) points out that the Gauguin myth has compelling appeal to men oriented more toward action than introspec-tion, men who in their middle years "would rather change their situa-tion than themselves" (p. 178), seeking a rebirth simply by traveling to a new land. She describes the painful reality Gauguin faced:

> In fact, there was nothing noble about Gauguin's life—and very little that was even pleasurable. He was actually a driven, self-destructive man who failed tragically in his flight into fantasy. And though he set sail for his tropical paradise with a wish to be "reborn," and redeemed, he actually spent the last years as an embittered exile who never gave up his desperate desire to be acclaimed by the society he supposedly despised. (p. 179)

Thus by comparing the myth and the reality of Gauguin's life, we illustrate the tendency to simplify and romanticize midlife crises and change in attempts to avoid the painful confrontation with the past that is an inevitable part of developmental progress in midlife.

Midlife Crisis, Transition, and Change

The term *midlife crisis* has become familiar because of its frequent use in popular books and on television talk shows. It has become a cliché, sometimes obscuring complex adult-developmental events or serious psychiatric illness, even severe depressive states. It behooves us to use the phrase carefully and with understanding. Is all change that occurs at midlife a "crisis?" The answer is no. For some individuals the feelings and events at midlife engender very little change. Others engage in a private, low-key self-questioning; a greater number seem to go through a more obvious transition. Some men and women, however, experience rather dramatic midlife change. As yet we do not have enough accurate normative data to determine how many people fall into those respective categories.

A true midlife crisis is a major and revolutionary turning point in one's life, involving changes in commitments to career and/or spouse and accompanied by significant and ongoing emotional turmoil for both the individual and others. In addition, the individual usually feels "unwell" in a context of uncertainty, anxiety, agitation, or depression. It is an upheaval of major proportions. One woman, on living through a midlife crisis, precipitated in part by divorce from her husband, described it as "the death of our family as we have known it."

The term *midlife transition* (Levinson, Darrow, Klein, Levinson, & McKee, 1978) probably has the greatest clinical utility at present because it includes aspects of crisis, process, and change. As described in Chapter 3, Levinson's intensive study of the life courses of 40 men demonstrated alternating periods of stability and transition throughout the life cycle. One such period was the midlife transition around ages 40 to 45. For a few the sense of change was slight and not particularly painful, a manageable transition. However, for approximately 80% the period of the early forties evoked tumultuous struggles within the self and with the external world.

Levinson described the state of mind of an individual in a midlife transition as a profound reappraisal which cannot be a cool, intellectual process. It must involve false starts, emotional turmoil, and despair. "Every genuine reappraisal must be agonizing, because it challenges the assumptions, illusions, and vested interests on which the existing structure is based" (p. 108).

PHENOMENOLOGY OF THE MIDLIFE TRANSITION

During the midlife transition an individual may confront himself (or herself) with some version of the following questions: "Is this really all there is to life? I want more out of life than this. Have I really accomplished anything? Where has my time gone? Is there anything that will really make me happy?" These are not necessarily the words of selfish, shallow, or unthinking individuals; they often emanate from responsible, successful, perceptive people. These people's anxiety and discomfort are complex and are frequently the summation of a variety of feelings and experiences that exert a common influence during midlife. For example:

Bodily changes, such as small changes in strength and endurance; slightly perceptible changes in skin and muscle tone; some decreases in energy and vigor; mild hearing or vision loss and slower reaction time; loss or graying of hair; or minor change in sexual interest with occasional impotence are reacted to with considerable anxiety by many people *because they symbolize time running out on them and stir feelings of anxiety about death.*

Changes in time perceptions are another midlife phenomenon, often experienced as "using up" the remaining hours of life at an ever-increasing pace (Greenleigh, 1974). "Total time left" is another concern of the middle-aged person. Neugarten (1975) describes a shift in thinking in middle age from "How long have I lived" to "How much time do I have left?" Total time left is brought clearly, sharply, and painfully to consciousness when a peer dies suddenly. Anxiety about death seems to be related to the striking sense of urgency that people in the midst of a midlife crisis experience.

Many individuals in our society, particularly men, reevaluate their work careers in midlife, sometimes, precipitating *career changes.* Work provides the primary answer to the question "Who am I?", and many men are primarily identified with their careers (Wilensky, 1960). For most men, career strivings are largely completed by the middle years; more highly educated men may continue to progress in their forties and fifties, but those who are less educated generally experience the beginning of a decline in their progress during their middle years and are seeking to hold on to the positions they have reached.

The discrepancy between career aspirations and achievements becomes a major issue in midlife. Until then one can dream of the career future and set flexible goals. In midlife the limitations of reality and time intrude on such dreams. Men may report a sense of obsolescence, particularly in regard to the challenge from younger men who come into the work arena highly valued for their youth and up-to-date knowledge. Reappraisal of career achievement is often only one facet of a serious questioning of one's life goals and values. Many "workaholics," compulsive workers to the exclusion of all else, experience midlife transformations.

Changes in marital relationship may occur during midlife, when many people experience a strong need to reassess their marriages. As Greenleigh (1974) points out, with children leaving home, the marriage and the meaning of the family are put to a test.

> Partners must assess their own relationship to determine whether it has the necessary ingredients to justify continuing their lives together . . . . Have the partners developed similarly and do they have enough in common? . . . If estranged, can they re-establish their relationship? (p. 64)

With concerns about physical aging and feelings of time running, the quest for the perfect partner is reignited, only to be dashed by an imperfect reality.

During midlife many individuals experience intense feelings of nostalgia for former lovers, questioning the current marital relationship and regretting seemingly missed opportunities for finding a perfect mate. If these feelings are intense enough they may lead to an active search and an extramarital affair. Not infrequently a husband or wife may turn to a younger individual in actuality or in fantasy, seeking a "fountain of youth" to restore and preserve one, or to magically undo concerns about bodily change, decreased time, and anxiety about death, as in the case report in Chapter 5.

Attitudes toward *children* can also become problematical at midlife. Although a good bit of attention has been given to adolescent turmoil, little has been studied or written about middle-age turmoil generated by parental response to adolescent children. In her novel *The War between the Tates* (1975), Allison Lurie describes feelings about the changes taking place in adolescent children:

> They were a happy family once, she thinks. Jeffrey and Matilda were beautiful, healthy babies; charming toddlers; intelligent, lively, affectionate children . . . .Then last year, when Jeffrey turned fourteen and Matilda twelve, they had begun to change; to grow rude, coarse, selfish, insolent, nasty, brutish and tall. It was as if she were keeping a boarding house in a

bad dream, and the children she had loved were turning into awful
lodgers—lodgers who paid no rent, whose leases could not be terminated.
They were awful at home and abroad; in company and alone; in the morning, the afternoon and the evening. (p. 12)

Middle age is truly a time of being *in the middle;* one is often responsible for the younger generation and not infrequently for the older
generation as well, so that *changes in parents* can also become an issue.
Neugarten and Datan (1974) quote from an interview with a particularly
perceptive woman:

> "It is as if there are two mirrors before me, each held at a partial angle.
> I see part of myself in my mother who is growing old and part of her in me.
> In the other mirror I see part of myself in my daughter. I have some dra-
> matic insights just from looking in those mirrors . . . a set of revelations that
> I suppose can come only when you are in the middle of three generations."
> (p. 383)

As elderly parents become less able to care for themselves, a role
reversal occurs for the middle-aged person. This may be a particularly
heavy burden if one is also dealing with adolescent children or the financial pressures of putting one or more children through college or
perhaps boarding a divorced daughter and her child (Sussman, 1977).
The facts that one's parents can no longer offer protection as they did
in childhood and indeed are reminders of one's own aging and death
often prompt painful intrapsychic adjustment and can lead to a sense
of crisis. For instance, the decision to institutionalize a decompensating
parent who needs constant physical care that the family cannot provide
threatens the existing psychic balance by engendering strong feelings
of guilt and shame and shattering the illusions of continuity that parents provide.

Social and financial change can be precipitated by the fact that,
whereas social insitutions used to convey a sense of permanence and
stability—in sharp contrast to the sense of impermanence and flux that
the middle-aged person experiences internally—they now appear to be
undergoing continual crises of integrity. Such changes have a direct effect on the equilibrium of the middle-aged and often contribute to and
heighten the sense of crisis. Take, for example, the divorce laws. Ten
or 15 years ago it was practically impossible to obtain a divorce in most
states. Today the pendulum has swung 180°, allowing rapid and in
some cases "do-it-yourself" divorce proceedings. The new laws support the fantasy of marital constancy only until "something better"
comes along.

Financial pressures are particularly acute in midlife and may contribute to feelings of tension and pressure. Real expenses reach a peak, along with a growing awareness of the need to plan for retirement. These demands create a conflict between wishes to spend money for present pleasure or to plan for a career change.

Case History. What follows is a case illustration of one man's rather tumultuous midlife crisis, transition, and ultimate transformation.

> The patient, J., was a 42-year-old man who walked into an outpatient psychiatric clinic after experiencing several days of upsurging rage, love, guilt, and anxiety associated with memories of childhood. In his words, "The rats were running," a reference to a flood of disturbing thoughts about his parents. For example, he visualized his father's death and a maternal reproach—"You killed him." That fantasy set off a string of thoughts about a communication barrier between himself and his parents and a failure to please them. Breaking through to them seemed urgent and hopeless. Vague suicidal ideation and the intensity of discomfort led to a desperate need for help before his business and social life were affected. J. saw his reaction as a reemergence of a problem that had begun four years before and had led to a year of psychotherapy at that time.
>
> *Psychiatric examination:* On the day of his first clinic visit J. was casually dressed, his hair disheveled. At times he raised his forearm across his forehead as if warding off an attack. Speech was pressured but thoughts were logical and coherent without evidence of bizarreness, delusions, or hallucinations. Completely oriented as to time, person, and place, J. demonstrated variation in mood from good humor to depression.
>
> *Family:* The patient's father was one of six from a middle-class family that contained both distinguished, accomplished individuals and several alcoholics. Father was described as a bright, stoic man who only told his son on three occasions that he loved him. J. felt he grew up without his father, who worked constantly and communicated by "a series of grunts." J.'s mother was from a poor family. Ashamed of her background, she "married up." A domineering woman, she controlled her husband and her family "like a field marshal." She expressed only anger and disappointment and encouraged her children to think of themselves as part of a respectable, hard-working family which would endure, successfully, under all circumstances. His parents' marriage appeared sterile and empty to J. Father rarely talked to mother either, possibly because for the past 10 years she had insisted on sleeping alone.
>
> J. admired his siblings, particularly the several who have become particularly successful, and he loved an older sister who took care of him during his early years, providing the warmth, affection, and nurturing that mother did not.
>
> *Some developmental highlights:* Born during the Depression, J. suspects that he was unwanted, yet his early memories place him in the center of attention. One vivid recollection was of his mother taking him into bed and patting him warmly on the back. Most pleasant remembrances focus

on his older sister caring for him. He recalled strong maternal reactions to his aggression, including verbal abuse and later, whippings that bordered on child abuse. J. relates his emergence as a practical joker to those beatings, feeling he had little other way to express his anger. Some of the "jokes" had serious consequences, such as dropping a heavy book on his brother's nose while his brother slept, digging holes and covering them with leaves and branches, and building a snowman around a fire hydrant and asking his friends to drive into it. Practical joking has continued to the present. Recently J. and his girl friend went separately to a bar; pretending to meet for the first time, they talked loudly about sex and left together.

J.'s childhood tendency to play tricks was accompanied by a vivid fantasy life. He described his clear recall of movies he had seen. He would lie in bed recreating the movie in exact detail, with himself as the main character. Although the intensity of such activity has diminished, it continues even today. For example, after a business meeting J. will relive it in his mind, changing events to determine a more successful outcome.

J.'s mother was prejudiced against certain ethnic and religious groups, a fact she hid in public. Although he never confronted her, J. was angered by his mother's stand and chose to retaliate. In high school he became the first non-Jewish member of a Jewish fraternity. Later in life he married the girl next door, a woman from an ethnic group and family disparaged by his mother.

In high school J. was interested in dramatics but avoided participating because he felt inferior to those students who were involved. Instead he joined other clubs but never assumed a position of leadership. J. had a number of friends of both sexes but did not have sexual intercourse at that time.

After high school J. spent four years in the service. He blames his father for that, since father took him to the recruiter when he could not make up his mind about college. During the enlistment he ma.ried a women with "the four V's—volatile, vicious, vituperative, and vivacious." He also went to night school and eventually earned a Master's degree and started a business. Despite his feelings about his wife, J. feels that his late twenties and thirties were good years. His business and marriage have prospered and he has fathered three children.

The crisis: When J. was 37 he found himself drawn to his 12-year-old son's religious and musical activities. Questions arising from his son's Sunday-school classes stimulated his own latent interest in religion. And he found himself drawn to and preoccupied with the lyrics of a popular song that stated that if a person didn't like what was in the world he could change it. *J. realized that he was an incomplete human being who had never expressed himself fully and who had the power to completely change his personality.*

He began to have regular family meetings during which he would tell his children his true feelings, including involvement in an extramarital affair. His wife objected to this practice and began to withdraw sexually. J. attempted to stay involved with his family but slowly began to lose self-confidence because he felt that his "new self," as he called it, and his new values could not survive his wife's criticisms and his own doubts. At that point J. began to experience a great fear of people and decided to leave his family. He recalled that his wife literally tore the shirt off his back in an attempt to restrain him as he went out the door. After providing financially for the family, J. disappeared into the woods, holing up in a mountain cabin. During the next two months he avoided all human contact, spending his time in the cabin deep in thought. On those occasions when he went out to get food he suspiciously covered his tracks so that his whereabouts would not be discovered.

His thoughts focused on childhood and his parents, for "the rats were running." He ranted and raved to himself, experiencing intense rage, guilt, and anxiety. After two months J. began going to a library where he would read theology and philosophy. He was struck by a statement that humans are different from other animals because they make love face to face, and also found himself intrigued by references to writings about people and the evolution of ideas. Thoughts of death were prominent during that time as J. "wrestled" with the concept of his own mortality. He felt "close to Christ" but also arrived at the intellectual decision that suicide was a viable choice for man. After six months J. became panicky and began psychotherapy, working on self-assertion, self-esteem, and reducing guilt; he remembers it as a rebuilding period.

J. returned home on Christmas Eve to a tearful reunion with his family. Over the course of the next year, despite the "absolute loss of a sense of humor," he reestablished his business, resumed a social life, and made a brief attempt to reconstitute his family. The latter was unsuccessful, followed by a divorce. J. left all of his material possessions to his wife, including their bank accounts.

Psychotherapy: J. entered into an intensive psychotherapeutic relationship with a conviction that this time he could come to grips with his feelings in a more definitive way and gain some peace and stability in his life. He worked particularly on his feelings about his parents and began to realize that in midlife the problem lay in his feelings about his parents, not in his parents themselves.

This man did have a true midlife crisis, according to our definition of it as a major and revolutionary turning point in life accompanied by significant emotional turmoil and changes in relation to family and career. His case illustrates clearly the reworking of the adult self as we described it in Chapter 5. J. begins to question his authenticity amid concerns about mortality. Neglected parts of his self seem to press for expression. His self-imposed retreat from others was, in part, an attempt at self-definition. In the midst of his narcissistic regression he ignores the needs of his family and cares only for himself, while grandly considering the philosophic questions of life including the religious meanings of life and death. Once reconstituted, J. returns to his family and discovers that his change makes it impossible for them to understand him and for him to need them. Like Moses, a changed person, a different self has come down from the mountain with a new plan of life. Over a period of several years he continues to work on tasks of separation–individuation by forging new relationships and a new career in an attempt to cast off aspects of the old or false self and make himself into a new man.

REFERENCES

Anderson, C. W. *Gauguin's paradise lost*. New York: Viking, 1971.

Greenleigh, L. Facing the challenge of change in middle age. *Geriatrics*, 1974, *29*, 61.

Levinson, D. J., Darrow, C. N., Klein, E. B., Levinson, M. H., & McKee, B. *The seasons of man's life*. New York: Alfred A. Knopf, 1978.

Lurie, A. *The war between the Tates*. New York: Warner, 1975.

Maugham, W. S. *The moon and sixpence*. New York: Doubleday, 1919.

Mayer, N. *The male mid-life crisis: Fresh starts after forty*. New York: Doubleday, 1978.

Neugarten, B. L. Adult personality: Toward a psychology of the life cycle. In W. C. Sze (Ed.), *The human life cycle*. New York: Jason Aronson, 1975, pp. 371–394.

Neugarten, B. L., & Datan, N. The middle years. In S. Arieti (Ed.), *American handbook of psychiatry*. New York: Basic Books, 1974, pp. 592–608.

Sussman, M. B. Family life of old people. In R. H. Binstock & E. Shanas (Eds.), *Handbook of aging and the social sciences*. New York: Van Nostrand Reinhold, 1977, pp. 218–243.

Wilensky, G. Careers, life styles, and social integration. *International Social Sciences Journal*, 1960, *12*, 553.

8

The Father at Midlife

CRISIS AND GROWTH OF PATERNAL IDENTITY

Fatherhood is more than a biological event or a psychological state limited to one phase of life; it is a complex developmental task that extends throughout the life cycle. *The basic concept of this chapter is that midlife (ages 35–55) is a particularly formative time in the evolution of paternal identity because of unique, phase-specific interaction between issues of midlife development in the father and adolescent development in his children.* It has long been apparent that middle-aged parents react strongly to their adolescent children. *However, that parental response is not only a reaction to the adolescent but also the result of equally (or more) salient developmental forces within the parent that are impinged upon by the adolescent is not generally understood.*

STUDIES ON THE DEVELOPMENT OF FATHERHOOD

As did Gurwitt (1976), we found the scarcity of psychodynamic studies on fathers and fatherhood surprising in view of ample recognition that becoming a father is an important psychological transition. As sparse as the literature on becoming a father is, studies concerning the *continuous evolution* of fatherhood are ever more rare.

The basis for this chapter is an article entitled "The Father at Midlife: Crisis and the Growth of Paternal Identity," appearing in an anthology on Fatherhood, edited by Stanley Cath, M.D., Allen Gurwitt, M.D., and John Munder Ross, Ph.D., to be published in 1982 by Little, Brown & Co.

Two significant commentaries illustrating the development, evolving nature of parenthood are those by Anthony and Benedek (1970) and by Pearson (1958). For Anthony and Benedek the biological root of fatherhood is in the instinctual drive for survival. Addressing herself specifically to the *developmental* role of fatherhood, Benedek (Anthony & Benedek, 1970) writes:

> The functions which represent fatherhood, fatherliness, and providing are parallel to motherhood, motherliness, and nurturing. Fatherhood and motherhood are complementary processes which evolve within the culturally established family structure to safeguard the physical and emotional development of the child. The role of the father within his family and his relationship with his children appear to be further removed from instinctual roots than those of the mother. . . . Fatherhood, i.e., the human male's role in procreation, has instinctual roots beyond the drive organization of mating behavior to include his function as provider and to develop the ties of fatherliness that make his relationship with his children a mutual developmental experience. (p. 167)

For example, as documented over and over again—by religious rite, custom, and socioeconomic organization—fathers search for immortality through their children, particularly their sons. Paternal identification with a son is immediate, for the father "can project into him the aspirations of his ego ideal, anticipating unconsciously his future self realization in his own son" (Anthony & Benedek, 1970, p. 172). The experience of being a father also powerfully influences the evolution of the adult personality when father engages dependency wishes stimulated by the inevitability of the adolescent's separation and further integrates childhood wishes to become like his own father.

Pearson (1958) is one of the few who have written specifically about dynamic conflicts and tensions within the middle-aged parent.

> As middle age comes on, the adult feels that he is passing his prime. He observes that his adolescent child is growing rapidly into a vigorous young adult with all his success ahead of him. He contrasts his lessening opportunities for success and his now rather static capacities with the budding development of his child, and unconsciously he feels envy. In his unconscious his child now seems to be a replica of his own parent; *and he begins to act to keep the child in his place* [italics added] just as he wanted to put his parents in *his* place when he was a child. The adolescent therefore has to struggle against these unconsciously motivated attitudes and actions of his parents and of other adults. (p. 21)

In the real and unconscious battle for power which ensues, the parent must, for the benefit of himself and his offspring, relinquish control of the adolescent's future. Pearson poetically describes an aspect of the conflict of generations as "two wounded narcissisms disliking each other" (p. 44). His advice to middle-aged parents is, "probably it is better for the adolescent if the parents close their eyes and lick their narcissistic wounds in silence, as much as they possibly can" (p. 44).

THE EFFECTS ON FATHERS OF THE REACTIVATION OF CHILDHOOD DEVELOPMENTAL THEMES AND CONFLICTS—THE OEDIPAL COMPLEX

Just as the experience of being a father influences the course of major adult-developmental tasks, so does it effect the *reengagement* of developmental issues and conflicts from childhood. Among the most prominent expressions of this intrapsychic process is the reactivation of the infantile oedipal complex, which we will now describe, and the separation–individuation process, which will be referred to later.

Pearson (1958) has described the *connection* between adult-developmental issues and the reactivation of oedipal conflicts.

> by the time an individual is in his late thirties or early forties—usually when his children are becoming adolescents—he begins to realize that he will probably never fulfill some of his postponed ideals. He perceives that he has already started on the downgrade toward old age and death, and this realization invigorates his fantasy of the reversal of generations. . . . The parent's realization that he is past the peak of his powers with so many goals never achieved makes him feel frustrated. *The frustration re-energizes the fantasy of the reversal of generations, and with it the envies, jealousies, and hatreds of the oedipus period.* (p. 177, italics added)

Father–Daughter Interactions

When the adolescent daughter begins to date, many oedipal feelings are stirred up in the middle-aged father by the introduction of a competitor, the boyfriend. Father's experience as a neglected outsider, observing a sexually charged relationship involving someone he loves, is similar to what he experienced as a child. Unlike the powerless child, the father may respond by attempting to dominate and control these dating relationships or he may involve himself in them inappropriately through excessive interest or teasing.

> A patient complained bitterly that his adolescent daughter was keeping him in the dark about her relationships with boyfriends. He felt excluded and betrayed. His feelings grew in intensity and disturbed him

since he recognized their inappropriateness and found it difficult to suppress powerful urges to repeatedly tease his daughter and her friends. In further associations the father described his anxious, angry response to his daughter's Halloween costume, which he described as "sexy and suggestive." Yet he wanted her to go to the party in question. Continued work revealed his phallic pride for having produced such a sexually stimulating woman and also his attraction to the young males who would vie for her attention. He described his admiration and envy of their youthful bodies and sexual energy which he magically hoped to capture for himself through his daughter.

Father and Son: Activity vs. Passivity, Strength vs. Weakness

As his teen-age son becomes more insistent on independence and autonomy, a father must relinquish some of his active control over the son's life. A necessary shift in the power balance between them occurs as the son tests, challenges, and eventually assumes mastery of his own life. This normative conflict ignites within the father feelings of rage, weakness, passivity, and helplessness in relation to another man who is important to him. We believe that this largely unconscious process is an inevitable part of the normal father's reaction to his maturing son and is responsible for precipitating a necessary developmental shift in the midlife parenting process which adds a new dimension to the role of fatherhood.

Accompanied by feelings of impotence, loss, dissolution, and resignation, the father must gradually abandon his role as parent of a young child. Because many gratifications of that role were related to the direct expression and sublimation of feelings of aggression through domination and control, the transition can be a painful one. Overreactions may take the form of attempts to reestablish dominance or, through reversal, an opposite situation may occur in which the father neglects the paternal limit-setting role, attempting to imitate the son rather than be his father.

It is our impression that the capacity for paternal *generativity* (Erikson, 1963) is determined in part by the resolution of this conflict. Through adult reworking, generativity is linked to masculinity as the passive, loving trends within a father's character are expressed by his care, unintrusive support, and facilitation of the emerging sexuality, independence, and separateness of late-adolescent and young-adult sons and daughters. Since the adolescent son is dealing with similar feelings and the same active-passive dichotomy, this generative responsiveness in the father often stimulates similar feelings in the son. For example, one adolescent voiced his strong dislike for one of his father's friends who was competitive and challenging but expressed affection for another whom he described as a "gentle giant."

For the father there is no final resolution of these issues, but a cyclic reengagement of them throughout adulthood. For instance, they peak again when the son chooses a partner—which may evoke feelings of jealousy and envy of, as one father put it, "his luscious young chick." In response father may compete for his son by offering advice, money, and companionship or, as in the case of one patient, by pleading (in a whining, helpless way) for his son's continued interest. Fantasies about the sexual life of the young couple may lead to conscious and unconscious identification with the son or possibly with his mate.

The nurturing, "feminine" side of the self can take on a new dimension, as it may have during the son's adolescence, and the result can be increased capacity for generativity now including the son's mate and eventually one's grandchildren as well. Continued self–object differentiation occurs throughout this process, leading to a more integrated, stronger sense of self which now includes new aspects of fatherhood—the roles of generative father and father-in-law.

Many of the basic concepts presented above are illustrated by the following clinical examples.

A 44-year-old father reported a wish to attend his teen-age son's parties and dances. Through a series of fantasies about his son's sexual activities it became clear that he unconsciously envied his young body and coveted his sexual prowess. As these wishes were interpreted in relation to his own aging process he began to experience intense feelings of pain, anger, and jealousy. When these feelings became conscious the patient acted by inappropriately attempting to restrict his son's dating and athletic activities. Only gradually was he able to assume a less intrusive, more supportive attitude. As treatment progressed, he became more aware of the futility of his search for youthful powers and its negative effects on family relationships, he began to appraise and appreciate his own considerable middle-age powers.

During his analysis, a 40-year-old business tycoon expressed a strong sense of worthlessness in relation to a powerful and very successful father. "My father was like a lion to me, the absolute king of the beasts." His own success, which surpassed his father's in many ways, had little effect on his sense of self-esteem. However, signs of healthy development in his latency-age and adolescent sons impressed him. Could he really be so bad if he was man enough and father enough to produce them? As he analyzed his overidealization and fear of his own father, he was able to engage his sons in a more relaxed, easy manner. To his surprise and delight they responded positively. "For the first time

I really feel like a somebody. I'm a hell of a better father than I thought."
As his children continued to develop they became living expressions of
his self-worth. The recognition of the importance of his adult feelings toward his sons was the key to the successful analysis of his unresolved
competitive "relationship" with his own father. The opportunity to work
through his adult conflicts about fatherhood was a factor in the lifting of
repression, thus allowing previously unavailable infantile sexual material, particularly in regard to his own father, to emerge. This integration
of adult experience and childhood conflict led to a more gratifying sense
of fatherhood and was reflected externally in a marked increase in parental effectiveness.

THE ADULT SELF AND FATHERHOOD

In Chapter 5 we explored the nature of the adult self, concentrating on a description of its emergence and characteristics and the narcissistic issues that underlie its development. Agreeing with Sutherland
(1978) and Saperstein and Gaines (1973), we saw considerable usefulness in conceptualizing a supraordinate self-system which mediates the
interaction of the person as a whole with his environment and is recognized as the final determiner of action. It is our impression that the
adult self evolves as the individual engages the major developmental
tasks of adulthood. Narcissistic gratifications and disappointments affect the evolution of the self as differences between idealizations and
realities become clear.

The experience of fatherhood is a determining influence on the
evolution of the adult self because it is such a central experience, full of
narcissistic gratification and disappointment. We are proposing here
that the representation of the concept, *father*, within the adult self undergoes evolution as the experience of fatherhood changes. For example, there is a considerable difference between the experience and intrapsychic representations of (a) being a 25-year-old father of a
three-year-old child, relating to a living father of 55, with a young wife
deeply involved in the care of her children, and (b) being a 45-year-old
father of late adolescents and young adults, relating to an aging or
dead father and preoccupied with the aging process in oneself and
one's wife. The experiences are so different and result in such altered
intrapsychic representation that perhaps the only thing remaining the
same is the name we give the experience.

The complex, evolving representation within the adult self is determined by many factors, among the most important of which are: (a)

experiences as a son—relating in the past and the present to one's own father and father substitutes (relatives, fathers of childhood friends); (b) experiences as a father—past and present experiences with one's own children and the children of others; and (c) related experiences— past and present experiences as a parent in concert with a spouse, as a sexual man, as a mentor and mentee.

PATERNAL RESPONSE TO SEPARATION AND LOSS

To illustrate our premise of the evolving nature of fatherhood we will use as an example the father's role in the separation–individuation process. We suggest that the father's role involvement in the second individuation in adolescence (Blos, 1967) is quantitatively and qualitatively different from his involvement in the infantile separation–individuation process (Mahler, 1975), not only because the child is different but also because father has changed as well. The developmental processes taking place between parents and adolescent children require a more basic and involved participation on the part of the father.

The psychobiological events of pregnancy (Bibring, 1959) prepare a mother for the extremely intimate, symbiotic tie with the child. Primarily a participant observer in the first individuation, the father serves as a buffer for both mother and child as they struggle against the powerful regressive pull toward symbiosis (Mahler, 1975). During the oedipal and latency years, father plays a role of increasing importance as a protector, provider, and example for his young children. By the onset of adolescence his position as a parent of equal importance to the mother is established in the minds of children, spouse, and the self.

The individuation of adolescent children, their movement from psychological and physical dependence to young adulthood, forces a reworking of the internal representation within the self of the father's role. He must transform the representation of himself as a protector and caretaker of young children and replace it with a new fathering identity as an interested facilitator, neither as necessary nor powerful.

This intrapsychic process is influenced by (1) paternal interaction with adolescent children around separation issues, (2) the father's reaction to separations and losses in his own life, and (3) his important involvement in the separation process occurring between mother and adolescent.

Some adolescents respond to the intrapsychic struggle over separation with an exaggerated, partly defensive, independent stance.

> One high-school senior insisted on handling all aspects of his application to college. He researched, filled out applications, and made a final decision entirely on his own, succeeding admirably in this task. His father's response to being so pointedly excluded was initially one of dismay and anger and only later of begrudging admiration. The appreciation of his son's adult competence and awareness that he would soon be leaving home precipitated a mourning reaction which gradually moved the father–son relationship toward greater equality and mutuality and redefined this man's understanding of himself as a parent.

Other adolescents struggle less against the separation process, and by so doing facilitate a gradual, less abrupt, but still painful intrapsychic loss and redefinition of fatherhood.

> One adolescent, very much his father's son, in addition to being a "straight-A" student, was also a companion, sharing mutual interests in academics, sports, and cars. Their planning together for college led to a gradual, smoother intrapsychic evolution for this particular father and also ignited intense feelings of grief over the loss of a son who was also a close friend.

The second major determinant of change in the representation of the concept *father* within the self is the reworking of separations from his own past, particularly during adolescence.

> One father commented that he had moved across the country from his family, and he feared his daughter would do the same. In anticipation of his daughter's departure for college, another man remembered his inability to express feelings about his leaving for college until a wrenching, tearful outburst of words and feelings at the airport. A third man, reacting to his son's aloofness, recalled homesickness when he himself had gone away from home for the first time at age 15. In each instance, further therapeutic work revealed connections between these adolescent experiences and their antecedents from earlier phases of development as well as their expression in the current reality with the fathers' adolescent children.

Another kind of dramatic, midlife separation experience is that forced by death. The death of a parent, particularly his father for a man, leads to a loosening of childhood introjects, forcing a reworking of separation issues, a reengagement of oedipal themes, and a new or altered caretaking relationship to a surviving, aging mother.

The painful disengagement of adolescent children from their mother and vice versa is a third major factor having a strong effect upon paternal identity. Because his relationship to his children is not based on the psychobiological experience of pregnancy and the powerful affective relationship of the first years of life, a father usually can observe the mother–child disengagement with some clarity and objectivity, even while he is engaged in a similar separation experience.

Although his role as a buffer between mother and infant was important during the first separation–individuation process, during adolescence it becomes central, even critical at times, since both mother and child may turn to him for help.

> While discussing his feelings about his adolescent daughter one father said, "You know, it was easier when she was a baby. I just left it all to my wife and went to work. But I can't do that now. My wife won't let me walk away, she needs me to help her deal with Amy, she insists on my help. Amy won't let me off the hook either. She comes to me more often than her mother." With a mixture of pride and annoyance he said, "You know I like it this way, but it sure as hell isn't easy."

> Another father reported his wife's anxiety when their son was late for breakfast while the family was on vacation. "He'll be here," he said, "stop worrying, he's 16 years old."

> A third father negotiated a more age-appropriate, realistic curfew for his 16-year-old daughter after mother and daughter had engaged in an intense verbal battle over the issue. Later he listened to his wife's sorrow and sense of impotence as she verbalized feelings about her daughter's independence and sexuality.

Such interactions help the father deal with his own sense of losing his children by allowing him to *actively* mediate similar feelings in his wife and children. They also lead to a redefinition of the marital relationship, which becomes more exposed as a dyad when children are gradually removed from the internal conceptions of husband–father and wife–mother.

INTIMATIONS OF GRANDPARENTHOOD

The awe and amazement that a father feels as he sees his adolescent children become physically, sexually, and psychologically mature bring with them the first awareness of the potential of grandfatherhood and considerable ambivalence about so inevitable a portent of aging and of eventual death. Anticipation of the event is a major stimulus which acts in the healthy father as a psychic organizer (Spitz, 1965). Increased awareness of aging becomes connected with the concept of grandfatherhood through compensatory fantasies of living on through grandchildren—a kind of genetic immortality through the narcissistically gratifying identification of one's characteristics in children and future grandchildren.

> One father obtained great pleasure from his late-adolescent son's obvious imitation of his shaving habits; the little boy who asked to use his razor at age three was now actually shaving just as he did. He was rather startled, somewhat pleased and also pained, by his growing awareness of a wish to have another little boy—his hoped-for grandson—copy his shaving habits.

As demonstrated by this example, the prospect of grandfatherhood brings with it the likelihood of recapturing the unambivalent admiration and love of young children, an attitude lost in the more realistic appraisal of older ones.

Another narcissistic gratification for the prospective grandfather is the reaffirmation of his sexuality through the fertility of his offspring. Their ability to produce children is a confirmation of his sexuality that takes on a special significance when physical retrogression and wanting sexual prowess may be problematic.

Last, but by no means least, the prospect of "spoiling" the grandchildren—the fantasized expression of impulses without restraint—is, through identification, applied to the self as well. Here is an outlet for expression of loving, nurturing, and gratifying impulses toward the self (through the grandchild) which comes in the life cycle at a time of increased frustration and deprivation through the loss of children and the sense of physical retrogression and aging.

REFERENCES

Anthony, E. J., & Benedek, T. *Parenthood*. Boston: Little, Brown, 1970.

Bibring, G. Some considerations of the psychological processes in pregnancy. *Psychoanalytic Study of the Child*, 1959, 14, 113.

Blos, P. The second individuation process of adolescence. *Psychoanalytic Study of the Child*, 1967, 22, 162.

Erikson, E. H. Eight ages of man. In *Childhood and society*. New York: W. W. Norton, 1963, pp. 247–269.

Gurwitt, A. Aspects of prospective fatherhood: A Core report. *Psychoanalytic Study of the Child*, 1976, 32, 237.

Mahler, M. S. Symbiosis and individuation: The psychological birth of the human infant. *Psychoanalytic Study of the Child*, 1975, 29, 89.

Pearson, G. *Adolescence and the conflict of generations*. New York: W. W. Norton, 1958.

Saperstein, J. L., & Gaines, J. Metapsychological considerations of the self. *International Journal of Psycho-Analysis*, 1973, *54*, 415.
Spitz, R. *The first year of life*. New York: International Universities Press, 1965.
Sutherland, J. *The self and personal object relations*. Unpublished manuscript, 1978.

9

Female Midlife Issues in Prose and Poetry

Although there are important similarities between the life courses of men and women, there are significant differences as well. In this chapter we explore aspects of these differences. If the study of midlife is a frontier, the study of women in midlife is the remotest outpost on that frontier because most major scientific studies to date have concentrated on men. However, important research results with regard to women are beginning to appear.

For instance, when the response of men and women to four common transitions of adult life (leaving home, starting a family, having an "empty nest," and retiring) were studied by Lowenthal, Thurner, and Cheroboga (1975), differences in adaptation were found to be more significant between the sexes than between older and younger members of the same sex. A second study, by Stewart (1977), who applied Levinson's theory of adult development (Levinson, Darrow, Klein, Levinson, & McKee, 1978), indicated that the development of women parallels that of men in the late teens and early twenties, but diverges considerably during the late twenties. By age 30, when both sexes have the opportunity to reassess their life structures, women have to "come to terms with issues of marriage and parenting in both a quantitatively and qualitatively different way than is the case for men" (p. 2). Stewart concluded that in our society, formation of a satisfactory early-adult life structure is more complex and difficult for women because, although

This chapter was written in collaboration with Susan L. Zuckerman, M.D., who was a senior medical student at the University of California at San Diego at the time.

traditional female goals are not valued as highly as those for men, women are nevertheless judged severely for not achieving them.

The material in this chapter is organized around four developmental themes of midlife: the body, object relations, work, and time and death.

THE FEMALE BODY

Although middle-aged men may still be seen as attractive and sexual, prevailing sociocultural views equate female sexual desirability with a youthful body. Simone de Beauvoir's (1974) prose puts the difference starkly:

> Whereas man grows old gradually, woman is suddenly deprived of her femininity; she is still relatively young when she loses the erotic attractiveness and the fertility which, in the view of society and in her own, provide the justification of her existence and her opportunity for happiness. With no future, she still has about one-half of her adult life to live. (p. 640)

Consequently, many middle-aged women experience more painful, more prolonged preoccupation with the physical signs of aging than do middle-aged men. Society's overevaluation of the youthful female body results in fears of being unsexed by age and losing love as a consequence.

The Hunger Artist

1

It's no use trying to find again
what it was like.
And the spectacle of it. The breasts
begin to go, skin
loosens under the chin.
You watch
an aging courtesan undress.

2

Him waiting, waiting as if
you never loved by night.
Long welts
of daylight, another bed.
To let it happen
easy as Eden, no wringing
of the mind, wrestle of leaves
to squeeze through.
His solemn arms, his room
not dark enough, your having
to be the way you are.

You fasten like things on a pond
to their own reflection.
Till he discovers that
you cannot play.

3

Remember your swimming
when a wave fell in.
Too stunned to fight the undertow,
you gave yourself up
dreaming to the pull.
When you lie down once more
in dangerous places
taking the fruit between your teeth,
there is always the light
thatched over another
who breathes beside you, entire,
strange to your wanting
even the least of what he was.

4

When plastic chairs in the kitchen
begin to crack, or fabric on the footstool wears
through to the stuffing,
or the sink falls slowly down
from the level of the formica counter
because water got in
under the unseen wood and is secretly
chewing it all away;
when you look in the mirror
after everyone leaves in the morning,
and the only sound is the thin hum
of the furnace, and suddenly
it stops, and the house begins to tick,
and you see the small wrinkles

under your lashes smudged
with mascara you never get off,
and you make a terrible smile
watching them deepen and lengthen
like thin lines raked in the sand
of a perfect Japanese garden;

you feel everything
being eaten from its surface.
Soon there will be no covers
and what is under
will be exposed, wasted
no longer able
to keep the flesh alive.

(Shirley Kaufman, 1973)

Bardwick (1971) and Rubin (1979) emphasize the importance of the adult woman's perception of herself as successful in her roles of wife and mother in resolving childhood and midlife ambivalence about sexuality and in overcoming fears associated with bodily change. Through the attainment of a happy love relationship with a man, a woman's unconscious anxieties about her sexuality may be diminished, for her ability to give and receive love and sexual gratification reassures and supports her against the guilt and fear associated with unresolved infantile sexual conflicts and wishes. Furthermore, the successful fulfillment of her reproductive role adds a new dimension of experience which facilitates a positive reworking of infantile feelings about the possession of an inferior or damaged genital. In her survey of middle-aged women, Rubin (1979) found that some had overcome a sense of sexual repression suffered since childhood, and viewed themselves as better sexual partners and felt sexually adequate for the first time in their lives. Such women are better able to resolve the conflicts about sexuality engendered by the physical changes at midlife (Bardwick, 1971). On the other hand, women whose husbands had rejected them had *more* fear about being sexually undesirable as a result of their age. For those who have not married or borne children, but who desire a marital and maternal role, signs of physical aging evoke fears of being unable to find a suitable mate before they are too old to attract men or bear children (Rubin, 1979).

For too long the menopause per se was considered the dominant factor in the psychology of middle-aged women, an entirely negative experience representing the loss of procreativity. We agree with Notman (1979) that psychological upheaval at midlife in women is not necessarily primarily menopausal, and to assume so can lead to inappropriate treatment of the supposed "deficiency disease" with estrogen supplements rather than helping the woman deal with what is in fact a normal progression leading to the next phase of her life. For women who have achieved security in their sexual identities, the sense of loss that accompanies cessation of the menses can be, and often is, transcended by a sense of excitement and increased enthusiasm for the future, a sense of being "restored to themselves" and to their own development.

OBJECT RELATIONS

The middle-aged woman must reshape her relationships with parents, now older and dependent, her middle-aged husband, now neither idealized nor exotic, and her children, who are establishing themselves as relatively independent individuals.

Parents

In relation to her parents a gradual role reversal is taking place. They no longer appear privileged and omnipotent; in all that she once envied—their physical size and strength, their sexuality, their reproductive ability, their independence and mastery of the world—it is likely that she now surpasses them. Feelings about this fact, which reactivate unresolved oedipal and preoedipal themes, may compromise her ability to respond to their increasing needs and build a new relationship with them.

Guilt and hostility elicited by this reversal in power between a daughter and her parents will be intensified if her struggle for independence and autonomy during adolescence and young adulthood was protracted and incompletely resolved. Whereas a son's rights to separation and autonomy are universally recognized and respected, similar needs have not been considered to be as important to a daughter's adult development. "A son's your son till he takes a wife; a daughter's your daughter all her life," goes the adage.

In general, women have more difficulty than men achieving a sense of autonomy or separation from their parents. According to Chodorow (1978), the prolonged dependency of women on their parents is grounded in the longer and more intense identification between a mother and her child of the same sex. A son is readily perceived as different and separate, but a daughter remains an extension of the mother's self for a longer time, and that relatively more intense symbiotic bond is difficult for the female child to break. Moreover, a mother is more aware of her heterosexual feelings toward her son than of her repressed homosexual feelings toward her daughter. The mother–son dyad moves rapidly toward a genitalized relationship which eventually requires the son to resolve his oedipal feelings by relinquishing his mother and identifying with his father. In contrast, the father–daughter dyad forms a more ambivalent love relationship because the girl's primary love object was her mother and in that sense her father is a substitute. This mother–daughter investment may be intensified by a father's greater commitment to his extrafamilial roles and less affective and active relationship to his children. So a daughter's resolution of preoedipal and oedipal feelings tends to be incomplete, and her vacillation between her parents is expressed by her ambivalence about achieving genuine autonomy.

During adolescence the girl again works through the triadic relationship with her parents by solidifying an attachment to her father and separating more completely from her mother, and then leaving her father to make a commitment to an extrafamilial love object. When blocks to this developmental process occur, the adolescent or young-adult woman is often unable to separate from her parents, and the power struggle continues, with hostile dependency, guilt, and vaguely sexualized love implicit in their relationship. Middle age can bring augmentation of the guilt as unconscious oedipal fantasies are reactivated, yet with that comes the opportunity for further resolution of the woman's conflicts over autonomy. The infantile bond to the parents is gradually weakened when adult love relationships gratify emotional and sexual needs, furthering the desexualization of love for the parents and rendering the aging parent(s) less necessary for emotional fulfillment.

The achievement of autonomy is also aided by becoming a parent. An intense investment in the mother–child dyad allows a reworking and a weakening of the infantile bond to her own mother, often in the face of less resistance because the new grandmother can reinvest in her grandchild the love no longer appropriate for her grown daughter (Bibring, 1961). The daughter's perception of herself as a mother in her own right diminishes the unconscious infantile envy of the maternal role and emphasizes the equality and mutuality that can exist between two adult women who are also mother and daughter.

Husband

Tolerance of ambivalence in a relationship is a prerequisite of the ability to genuinely care for another and commit oneself to a mate (Kernberg, 1974). With increased tolerance for ambivalent feelings in midlife, the previously idealized lover can be perceived more realistically and the earlier idealization transformed into mature devotion. The following poem by Dianne DiPrima (1975) illustrates her commitment to and identification with her husband and his ideal of himself, as well as her acceptance of him as he is.

Quartz Light

the man
you wish to be
are not
I love
as I love you
wishing to be
the man

as I love
you who are
you stand so straight
your hand on my arm
a tremulousness

In conjunction with renunciation of other possible loves, a couple continually redefines their own ideals to meet unfulfilled or changing needs and goals, simultaneously gaining heightened appreciation of the valuable qualities in one another and their relationship. In a second poem, DiPrima (1975) expresses qualities that Kernberg (1974) finds in a mature love relationship, such as tolerance for ambivalence, identification, empathy, and concern for the beloved, as well as commitment to the evolving relationship.

Poem in Praise of my Husband (Taos)

I suppose it hasn't been easy living with me either,
with my piques, and ups and downs, my need for privacy
leo pride and weeping in bed when you're trying to sleep
and you, interrupting me in the middle of a thousand poems
did I call the insurance people? the time you stopped a poem
in the middle of our drive over the nebraska hills and
into colorado, odetta singing, the whole world singing in me
the triumph of our revolution in the air
me about to get that down, and you
you saying something about the carburetor
so that it all went away

but we cling to each other
as if each thought the other was a raft
and he adrift alone, as in this mud house
not big enough, the walls dusting down around us, a fine dust rain
counteracting the good, high air, and stuffing our nostrils

we hang our pictures of the several worlds;
new york collage, and san francisco posters,
set out our japanese dishes, chinese knives
hammer small indian marriage cloths into the adobe
we stumble thru silence into each other's gut

blundering thru from one wrong place to the next
like kids who snuck out to play on a boat at night
And the boat slipped from its moorings, and they look at the stars
about which they know nothing, to find out
where they are going.

Although marital stability is promoted by commitment and deepened by concern for one's partner and shared experiences over time, there are no guarantees; for if the original partner fails to remain compatible with maturing ideals, values, and needs, the relationship may flounder. This fact is especially relevant today when, as Stewart (1977) notes, many women who have maintained traditional roles find at midlife that they want more egalitarian relationships with their husbands as well as extrafamilial careers. Such major changes in the woman's view of herself, her partner, and their relationship provoke stress; and the preservation of marital stability, as noted by Nadelson, Polansky, and Mathews (1978), depends on the couple's ability to function as a unit in resolving the consequences of their different rates and directions of growth and change.

When the marital relationship survives the developmental pitfalls of midlife, it provides one means for further growth, resolution, and pleasure. For instance, Binstock (1973) suggests that as the woman's identity and ego boundaries are more sharply defined through her sexual and affective experiences in a mature relationship, the remnants of her fear of fusion and loss of individuality are mitigated, and reconfirmation of the physical and psychic boundaries allows an ever increasingly intimate relationship with her partner.

After Love

Afterwards, the compromise.
Bodies resume their boundaries

These legs, for instance, mine
your arms take you back in.

Spoons of our fingers, lips
admit their ownership.

The bedding yawns, a door
blows aimlessly ajar

and overhead, a plane
sing songs coming down.

Nothing is changed, except
there was a moment when

the wolf, the mongering wolf
who stands outside the self

lay lightly down and slept.

(Maxine Kumin, 1973)

In Kernberg's (1974) view, the resolution of infantile sexual conflicts enables the woman to come to terms with both her heterosexual and homosexual identifications; that is, to be able to identify with male sexuality and the male sex role as well as experience a fuller sense of her own sexual identity. Empathizing and identifying with her partner's sexuality and their past experiences together, she works to increase her own enjoyment of love and sex, in the process experiencing a deepening of their relationship which includes an intense specificity.

First Things

I can't name love now
without naming its object—
that is the final measure
of those flintspark years
when one believed
one's flash innate.
Today I swear
only in the sun's eye
do I take fire.

(Adrienne Rich, 1967)

Song: Remembering Movies

remembering movies love
remembering songs
remembering the scenes and flashes of your life
given to me as we lay dreaming
giving dreams
in the sharp flashes of light
raining from the scenes of your life
the faithless stories, adventures, discovery
sexuality opening range after range
and the sharp music driven forever into my life
I sing the movies of your life
the sequences cut in rhythms of collision
rhythms of linkage, love,
I sing the songs.

(Muriel Rukeyser, 1976)

Such fulfillment allays fears of becoming sexually undesirable as a result of aging, attenuates preoccupation with physical imperfections (Rubin, 1979), and leads to increased acceptance of the body as it is.

Poem in Which My Legs Are Accepted

Legs!
How we have suffered each other,
never meeting the standards of magazines or official measurements.

I have hung you from trapezes,
    sat you on wooden rollers,
      pushed and pulled you with the anxiety of taffy,
and still, you are yourselves!

Most obvious imperfection, blight on my fantasy life,
strong,
plump,
never to be skinny
or even hinting of the svelte beauties in history books or
    Sears catalogues.

Here you are—solid, fleshy and
white as when I first noticed you, sitting on the toilet
    spread softly over the wooden seat,
having been with me only twelve years,
    yet
as obvious as the legs of my thirty-year old gym teacher.

Legs!
O that was the year we did acrobatics in the annual gym show.
How you split for me!
    One-handed cartwheels
    from this end of the gymnasium to the other,
    ending in double splits,
legs you flashed in blue rayon slacks my mother bought
                for the occasion
and tho you were confidently swinging along
the rest of me blushed at the sound of clapping.

Legs!
How I have worried about you, not able to hide you,
embarrassed at beaches, in high school
        when the cheerleaders' slim brown legs
           spread all over
           the sand
           with the perfection
           of bamboo
I hated you, and still you have never given out on me.

With you
I have risen to the top of blue waves,
with you
I have carried food home as a loving gift

> when my arms began un-
> jelling like madrilenne.
> Legs, you are a pillow
> white and plentiful with feathers for his wild head,
> You are the endless scenery
> behind the tense sinewy elegance of his two dark legs.
> You welcome him joyfully
> and dance.
> And you will be the locks in a new canal between continents.
> The ship of life will push out of you
> and rejoice
> in the whiteness,
> in the first floating and rising of water.
>
> (Kathleen Fraser, 1973)

When all goes well this deepening of ego and sexual identities and trust in their boundaries allow two adults to enjoy mutual dependency and support rather than feel the insecurity and uncertainty that attends any immature relationship. The resulting *authentic intimacy*, a core experience of midlife, brings a mature joy and fulfillment only possible at that developmental stage.

Mother–Daughter Relationship

The middle-aged woman must accept her adolescent daughter's developing womanhood, independence, and individuality and establish a more distant yet supportive relationship with her. This requires a working through of feelings of competition and jealousy as well as an acceptance of filial rejection of maternal values. Because of changing sociocultural attitudes, daughters today have greater sexual freedom and more options with respect to future familial and extrafamilial roles than their mothers had as adolescents or even as adults. Just when she may be recognizing the limits imposed on her own opportunities by society, husband, children, and the passage of time, the middle-aged mother finds herself confronted with her daughter's present and future opportunities to express and develop all aspects of her personality. This realization evokes memories of abandoned adolescent dreams and fantasies and heightens the sense of loss and lack of fulfillment with respect to her own aspirations.

Moreover, her daughter's increasing separation and need to individuate, superimposed on internalized sociocultural attitudes about women, may be experienced as a rejection of herself and her values.

Deutsch (1944) observed that often the adolescent girl turns from her mother as a role model and forms a more intimate relationship with a peer, female teacher, or relative. Admiration and affection for those women, combined with an aloof and critical attitude toward mother, may make the mother feel devalued and replaced as an important and respected person in her daughter's life.

Such feelings can be resolved through a process of identification in which she shares in her daughter's future happiness, which represents the potential and opportunities the mother no longer has. In that way the middle-aged woman can gain a sense of immortality and repair her narcissistic injuries as she facilitates the passage of her daughter and herself into new periods of their lives, as in the following poem by Anne Sexton (1966) addressed to a daughter entering adolescence:

Little Girl, My Stringbean, My Lovely Woman

My daughter, at eleven
(almost twelve), is like a garden.

Oh, darling! Born in that sweet birthday suit
and having owned it and known it for so long,
now you must watch high noon enter—
noon, that ghost hour.
Oh, funny little girl—this one under a blueberry sky,
this one! How can I say that I've known
just what you know and just where you are?

It's not a strange place, this odd home
where your face sits in my hand
so full of distance,
so full of its immediate fever.
The summer has seized you,
as when, last month in Amalfi, I saw
lemons as large as your desk-side globe—
that miniature map of the world—
and I could mention, too,
the market stalls of mushrooms
and garlic buds all engorged.
Or I think even of the orchard next door,
where the berries are done
and the apples are beginning to swell.
And once, with our first backyard,
I remember I planted an acre of yellow beans
we couldn't eat.

Oh, little girl,
my stringbean,
how do you grow?
You grow this way.
You are too many to eat.

I hear
as in a dream
the conversation of the old wives
speaking of *womanhood*.
I remember that I heard nothing myself.
I was alone.
I waited like a target.

Let high noon enter—
the hour of the ghosts.
Once the Romans believed
that noon was the ghost hour,
and I can believe it, too,
under startling sun,
and someday they will come to you,
someday, men bare to the waist, young Romans
at noon where they belong,
with ladders and hammers
while no one sleeps.

But before they enter
I will have said,
Your bones are lovely,
and before their strange hands
there was always this hand that formed.

Oh, darling, let your body in,
let it tie you in,
in comfort.
What I want to say, Linda,
is that women are born twice.

If I could have watched you grow
as a magical mother might,
if I could have seen through my magical transparent belly,
there would have been such ripening within:
your embryo,
the seed taking on its own,
life clapping the bedpost,
bones from the pond,
thumbs and two mysterious eyes,
the awfully human head,
the heart jumping like a puppy,
the important lungs,
the becoming—
while it becomes!
as it does now,
a world of its own,
a delicate place.

I say hello to such shakes and knockings and high jinks,
such music, such sprouts,
such dancing-mad-bears of music,
such necessary sugar,

such goings-on!

Oh, little girl,
my stringbean,
how do you grow?
You grow this way.
You are too many to eat.

What I want to say, Linda,
is that there is nothing in your body that lies.
All that is new is telling the truth.
I'm here, that somebody else,
an old tree in the background.
Darling,
stand still at your door,
sure of yourself, a white stone, a good stone—
as exceptional as laughter
you will strike fire,
that new thing!

The Mother–Son Relationship

A mother's ability to modify her relationship with an adolescent son depends, in part, on the ability to accept his increasing independence, to repress her sexual impulses toward him, and to overcome jealousy of his extrafamilial life, particularly his girl friends. The son's drive for separateness from his mother evokes many feelings including loss and abandonment, pride in his accomplishment and growth, and, as with the daughter, an identification with and envy of his future. Her sexual feelings for him are powerful and stimulating and result in a complicated response toward his girl friends.

The strength of those feelings, and their lack of resolution, are powerfully demonstrated by the following poem.

Two Sons

Where and to whom
you are married I can only guess
in my piecemeal fashion. I grow old on my bitterness.

On the unique occasion
of your two sudden wedding days
I open some cheap wine, a tin of lobster and mayonnaise.
I sit in an old lady's room
where families used to feast
where the wind blows in like soot from north-northeast

Both of you monopolized
with no real forwarding address
except for two silly postcards, you bothered to send home,

one of them written in grease
as you undid her dress
in Mexico, the other airmailed to Boston from Rome

just before the small ceremony
at the American Church
Both of you made of my cooking, those suppers of starch

and beef, and with my library,
my medicine, my bath water,
both sinking into small brown pools like muddy otters!

You make a toast for tomorrow
and smash the cup,
letting false women lap the dish I had to fatten up.

When you come back I'll buy
a wig of yellow hair;
I'll squat in a new red dress: I'll be playing solitaire
on the kitchen floor.
Yes . . . I'll gather myself in
like cut flowers and ask you how you are and where you've been.

(Anne Sexton, 1966)

On the other hand, a woman may deal with her anger, jealousy, and rivalry in a more constructive manner, through identification with her son's new life, by forming a close relationship with her daughter-in-law, and by anticipating the experience of grandmotherhood. That new developmental experience provides another opportunity to engage maternal feelings, to reexperience the awe of childhood from within the confines of a close, loving relationship, and to deal with wishes for immortality by incorporating the youth of the grandchild into the self.

Although the discussion to this point has emphasized the loss that mothers feel as their children separate, it is important to recognize that as only one of the feelings involved. Women also experience the separation from grown children as a developmental stimulus and as a source of pleasure and relief. In fact, given the complexity of the dynamic issues involved in appropriate separation from one's children in midlife, it becomes as difficult to maintain the myth of the empty-nest syndrome as to maintain the myth that the menopause explains all. Rubin (1979) found that most of her 160 subjects (women from 35 to 44, graduates of high school or college, and of moderate economic means) had given up pursuit of their own jobs or careers to devote themselves full-time to the family for about 10 years. Despite that dedication, Rubin did not find a simple cause-and-effect relationship between their children leaving home and maternal depression. In many women she discovered instead a decided sense of relief and anticipation. To Rubin's thinking, then, the crisis at that period centers not around the children leaving but around the necessity to develop alternatives to mothering. Whereas a man may prepare for one career and pursue it through retirement, a woman may need to master three careers: a first career, then motherhood, then a third career. So anxiety about what to do after the children leave contributes to and may be a central component of the crisis for many women. One of Rubin's subjects spells it out:

> "What has been and still is traumatic is trying to find the thing I want to do, and being able to pursue it to a successful conclusion . . . it's hard to make the kind of commitment that real success requires. I'm afraid of what it'll do to my marriage, and also to the rest of my life. And I suppose I'm afraid to really try and fail. But that's the stuff that's so hard and painful right now; it's not knowing what I'll be doing, or even that I *can* do. And from 45 to 75 is a lot of years if I don't have something useful to do." (pp. 39–40)

Work

"No other technique for the conduct of life attaches the individual so firmly to reality as laying emphasis on work," said Freud (1930), "for his work at least gives him a secure place in portion of reality, in the human community" (p. 80). Work, he noted, is an extremely essential and complex function which gives expression to erotic, narcissistic, and aggressive needs and impulses. Because society tends to relate achievement and success predominantly to paid employment, many women discount the value of their familial role. Influenced by economic necessity; by the feminist movement, which has popularized the attitude that women can and should pursue work-related personal goals; and by intrapsychic pressures, women are entering the paid work force in ever-increasing numbers. Bardwick (1971) and Mogul (1979) both point out, however, that the result is a disappointment for many because of idealized notions of the work situation, unrealistic expectations about the opportunities available, and significant age and sex discrimination.

Work outside the home is potentially more conflict-laden for women than for men. Furthermore, the middle-aged woman's motivation to work is psychologically complex, based on desires to realize unfulfilled goals and values, to achieve increased status and self-esteem from a socioculturally valued role, and to adapt to and deal with age-related issues. These intrapsychic forces exist in the context of a rapidly changing, fluctuating, but increasingly accepting social attitude toward working women.

The result of the intermixture of these personal and cultural factors can be emotional upheaval, doubt, depression, and a sense of being unfulfilled.

Housewife

So I live inside my wedding ring,
Beneath its arch,
Multiplying the tables of my days,
Rehearsing the lessons of this dish, that sleeve,
Wanting the book that no one wrote,
Loving my husband, my children, my house,
With this pain in my jaw,
Wanting to go.

Do others feel like this? Where do they go?

(Susan Fromberg Schaeffer, 1974)

Thoughts on the Education of Daughters

"To have in this uncertain world some stay
which cannot be undermined, is
of the utmost consequence."
                              Thus wrote
a woman, partly brave and partly good,
who fought with what she partly understood.
Few men about her would or could do more,
hence she was labelled harpy, shrew and whore.

(Adrienne Rich, 1967)

The conflicted feelings arising from simultaneous wishes for success and fear of failure, and the distorted emphasis on women's sexual identity to the exclusion of her total identity are expressed by Erica Jong (1973):

Alcestis on the Poetry Circuit

The best slave
does not need to be beaten
She beats herself.

. . . .

She should mistrust herself
in everything but love
She should choose passionately
& badly.
She should feel lost as a dog
without her master.

She should refer all moral questions
to her mirror.
She should fall in love with a cossack
or a poet.
. . . .
Though she is quick to learn
& admittedly clever,
her natural doubt of herself
should make her so weak
that she dabbles brilliantly
in half a dozen talents
& thus embellishes
but does not change
our life.

If she's an artist
& comes close to genius
the very fact of her gift
should cause her such pain
that she will take her own life
rather than best us.

& after she dies, we will cry
& make her a saint.

(pp. 25–26)

The conflicts attending work may be less intense for women who hold positions of authority over other women or children rather than men, because both men and women accord greater prestige to success in male-dominated fields. Where male domination exists it tends to be self-perpetuating because of the absence of female role models and mentors. Sheehy (1974) observed that professional women have fewer mentor relationships than men; those that exist are often unsatisfactory, sometimes even destructive to the consolidation of professional identity. If the only available mentor is a man, two dangers exist: he may attempt to exploit his protégée sexually, or he may assume a paternalistic stance. Either way the mentee's embryonic professional identity is compromised.

Work and Loved Ones

A commitment to work affects a woman's relationships with her parents, husband, and children. Resumption of work may unconsciously represent repudiation of her own *mother's* values, or a triumph over her (Applegarth, 1977). Through assuming a work role she may battle unconsciously with her mother for her father's approbation, or compete with *father* himself—all during a period when it is especially important to consolidate positive relationships with aging parents.

Many women experience hostility and resentment from their *husbands* in relation to work. After overcoming her own inhibitions and fears, a woman may receive tenuous support from a husband who is threatened by an erosion of dominance as the couple moves toward a more egalitarian relationship (Rubin, 1979). If her husband's work is considered to be primary and she organizes her own life and work around that, emotional consequences are sure to follow.

Since adolescent and young-adult children are struggling to separate from mother and establish their own identities, they may react negatively to her ambition and assertiveness, fearing that she is rejecting, punishing, or competing with them. Rivalry may be especially keen between mother and daughter, particularly if the daughter is establishing her identity through a traditional family role. On the other hand, if the daughter is also pursuing a career, she may feel that her mother is undercutting her achievements in that sphere. In any event, confusion and ambivalence about her new goals must be faced as the working, middle-aged mother restructures her life and redefines her relationships.

TIME AND DEATH

Perhaps the most fundamental task of midlife is to resolve the conflict between the unconscious sense of timelessness, infinite time, immortality, and onmipotence and the ego's sense of time, time limitations, personal vulnerability, and death. "In the unconscious everyone is convinced of his own immortality . . . .There is nothing in the id that corresponds to the idea of time; and there is no recognition of the passage of time" said Freud (1915, p. 289).

Jacques (1965) feels that the resolution of the midlife crisis and the achievement of mature adulthood are based on the acceptance of the inevitability of one's own death; Neugarten (1973) sees the central psychological task of middle age as mastery of the use of time. For both men and women, resolution of conflicting internal representations of time is influenced by object relations, physical changes in oneself and others, and sociocultural attitudes. Loosening or lost familial ties are generally felt more irtensely in midlife by women than by men, for women are usually involved more intimately with their children and have been more emotionally dependent on their parents. As we have noted, also, sociocultural emphasis on the sexual and reproductive roles and the desirability of a youthful appearance increase the fear and the significance of the losses associated with physical aging and menopause. Women who have compromised or sacrificed personal goals in response to external or internal pressures feel even more acutely such losses of the ideal self around midlife.

In particular, the changing object relations of midlife, punctuated by the separation of adolescent and young-adult children and the eventual death of her parents, deeply influence a woman's attitudes toward personal death. Mahler (1973) notes that during middle age a woman may experience as a loss akin to death the increasing distance from her children. To the extent that a woman has centered her life around her children and has incorporated the notion that her worth and purpose as an individual are related primarily to the maternal role, she may experience intense feelings of loss and a sense that her useful life is over. The failing health and death of parents further emphasizes the passage of time and the inevitability of death, for, as Freud (1915) stated, one learns about personal death by experiencing the loss of a part of the self when loved ones die.

Somatic aging speaks of death as the woman struggles with accepting the loss of her youthful body.

Age

I grow old in the house of my body
Wicker rockers tilt in my eyes

Pink camelias grow in my hair
Though I clip them and clip them

They are whispering to my pleated breasts
and my thighs, you are *young, young, young*.

(Susan Fromberg Schaeffer, 1974)

Women are more pressured and restricted than men by what Neugarten (1973) terms a socially defined sense of time, or a sense of the temporal appropriateness of major events in life. Such socially defined standards are generally based on the male life cycle, wherein by midlife one is expected to be firmly established in a career. Women who have devoted their early adulthood to establishing a family and who then desire a career view themselves and are viewed by others as out of synchrony with appropriate temporal standards. Stewart (1977) found that married women from 31 to 40 who had no career or extrafamilial goals showed an increased desire for extrafamilial commitments and independence from their husbands, sometimes at the expense of marital stability. On the other hand, unmarried women who had established themselves in a career felt pressured to marry by age 30 because of a growing pressure to have a child before it was too late.

Because of the wish to achieve all and the inability to do so, the middle years are characterized by a jarring reappraisal of what has been accomplished and what is possible.

Letter to John Wieners (on his 37th birthday)

Dear John, we are old now
& we have not
any of us, done whatever it was
we set out to do, in the glow of the
blue-white crystals, in the shadow
of the black leather drapes. But we have
done something, drawn some line
across the sky, jetstream, a monument
to our bewilderment, our hope
at a black crossroads that glistened
like jet in our hands, a deathrite we saw thru
for the pale numberless children whose names
I no longer remember, for a planet that flashed
color once, red plumage, there is a taste
in my mouth like the taste of the dawn, salt taste
of dirty, weary bodies falling out
across the room, the high excitement
ebbed, look, I'll dip my hands
in that milky way we made, this icy juice
that burns me to the bone, can you call it
forgiveness, or love?

(Dianne DiPrima, 1975)

Gradually, as the woman struggles with her limitations and her mortality, a sense of resolution and peace emerges.

At Majority

When you are old and beautiful,
And things most difficult are done,
There will be few who can recall
Your face that I see ravaged now
By youth and its oppressive work.

Your look will hold their wondering looks
Grave as Cordelia's at the last,
Neither rancor at the past
Nor to upbraid the coming time.
For you will be at peace with time.

But now a daily warfare takes
Its toll of tenderness in you,
And you must live like captains who
Wait out the hour before the charge—
Fearful, and yet impatient too.

Yet someday this will have an end,
All choices made or choice resigned,
And in your face the literal eye
Trace little of your history,
Nor ever piece the tale entire

Of villages that had to burn
And playgrounds of the will destroyed
Before you could be safe from time
And gather in your brow and air
The stillness of antiquity.

(Adrienne Rich, 1967)

The midlife confrontation with goals unmet, choices not made, and aging brings with it mature insight into the ways death is viewed in childhood and adulthood and a bittersweet understanding of the second half of the life cycle.

Childhood Is the Kingdom Where Nobody Dies

Childhood is not from birth to a certain age and at a certain age
The child is grown, and puts away childish things.
Childhood is the kingdom where nobody dies.

Nobody that matters, that is. Distant relatives of course
Die, whom one never has seen or has seen for an hour,
And they gave one candy in a pink-and-green striped bag, or a jack-knife,
And went away, and cannot really be said to have lived at all.
And cats die. They lie on the floor and lash their tails,
And their reticent fur is suddenly all in motion
With fleas that one never knew were there,
Polished and brown, knowing all there is to know,
Trekking off into the living world.
You fetch a shoe-box, but it's much too small, because she won't curl up now;
So you find a bigger box, and bury her in the yard, and weep.

But you do not wake up a month from then, two months,
A year from then, two years, in the middle of the night
And weep, with your knuckles in your mouth, and say Oh, God! Oh God!
Childhood is the kingdom where nobody dies that matters—mothers and
    fathers don't die.

And if you have said, "For heaven's sake, must you always be kissing
    a person?"
Or, "I do wish to gracious you'd stop tapping on the window with your
thimble!"

Tomorrow, or even the day after tomorrow if you're busy having fun,
Is plenty of time to say, "I'm sorry, mother,"

To be grown up is to sit at the table with people who have died,
    who neither listen nor speak;
Who do not drink their tea, though they always said
Tea was such comfort.

Run down into the cellar and bring up the last jar of raspberries;
    they are not tempted.
Flatter them, ask them what was it they said exactly
That time, to the bishop, or to the overseer, or to Mrs. Mason;
They are not taken in.
Shout at them, get red in the face, rise,
Drag them up out of their chairs by their stiff shoulders and shake
    them and yell at them;
They are not startled, they are not even embarrassed; they slide
    back into their chairs.

Your tea is cold now.
You drink it standing up,
And leave the house.

                    (Edna St. Vincent Millay, 1956)

The Leaf and the Tree

When will you learn, my self, to be
A dying leaf on a living tree?
Budding, swelling, growing strong,
Wearing green, but not for long,
Drawing sustenance from air,
That other leaves, and you not there,
May bud, and at the autumn's call
Wearing russet, ready to fall?

Has not this trunk a deed to do
Unguessed by small and tremulous you?
Shall not these branches in the end
To wisdom and the truth ascend?
And the great lightning plunging by
Look sidewise with a golden eye
To glimpse a tree so tall and proud
It sheds its leaves upon a cloud?

Here, I think, is the heart's grief;
The tree, no mightier than the leaf,
Makes firm its root and spreads its crown
And stands; but in the end comes down.

That airy top no boy could climb
Is trodden in a little time
By cattle on their way to drink.
The fluttering thoughts a leaf can think,
That hears the wind and waits its turn,
Have taught it all a tree can learn.

Time can make soft that iron wood.
The tallest trunk that ever stood,
In time, without a dream to keep,
Crawls in beside the root to sleep.

(Edna St. Vincent Millay, 1956)

REFERENCES

Applegarth, A. Some observations of work inhibitions in women. In H. Blum (Ed), *Female psychology*. New York: International Universities Press, 1977, pp. 257–268.

Bardwick, J. *Psychology of women*. New York: Harper & Row, 1971.

Bibring, S. A study of the psychological processes in pregnancy and the earliest mother-child relationship. *Psychoanalytic Study of the Child*, 1961, *16*, 9.

Binstock, W. On the two forms of intimacy. *Journal of the American Psychoanalytic Association*, 1973, *21*, 93.

Chodorow, N. *Mothering*. Berkeley: University of California Press, 1978.

de Beauvoir, S. *The second sex*. New York: Vintage Books, 1974.

Deutsch, H. *The psychology of women* (Vol. 1). New York: Grune & Stratton, 1944.

DiPrima, D. *Selected poems: 1956–1975*. Plainsfield, Vt.: North Atlantic Books, 1975, pp. 170, 190, 251.

Fraser, K. Poem in which my legs are accepted. In L. Chester & S. Barba (Eds.), *Rising tides: 20th century American women poets*. New York: Washington Square Press, 1973, pp. 297–298.

Freud, S. *Thoughts for the times on war and death*, Standard edition, 14:273. London: Hogarth Press, 1915.

Freud, S. *Civilization and its discontents*, Standard edition, 21:59. London: Hogarth Press, 1930.

Jacques, E. Death and the mid-life crisis. *International Journal of Psycho-Analysis*, 1965, *46*, 602.

Jong, E. *Half-Lives*. New York: Holt, Rinehart & Winston, 1973, pp. 25–26.

Kaufman, S. The hunger artist. In L. Chester & S. Barba (Eds.), *Rising tides: 20th century American women poets*. New York: Washington Square Press, 1973, pp. 127–129.

Kernberg, O. Mature love: Prerequisites and characteristics. *Journal of American Psychoanalytic Association*, 1974, *22*, 743.

Kumin, M. After love. In L. Chester & S. Barba (Eds.), *Rising tides: 20th century American women poets*. New York: Washington Square Press, 1973, p. 163.

Levinson, D. J., Darrow, C. N., Klein, E. B., Levinson, M. H., & McKee, B. *The seasons of a man's life*. New York: Alfred A. Knopf, 1978.

Lowenthal, M. F., Thurner, M., & Cheroboga, D. *Four stages of life: A comparative study of men and women facing transitions*. San Francisco: Jossey-Bass, 1975.

Mahler, M. In Winestine, M. (Reporter), The experience of separation–individuation . . . through the course of life: Infancy and childhood (Panel report). *Journal of the American Psychoanalytic Association*, 1973, *21*, 125.

Millay, E. S. *Collected Poems.* New York: Harper & Row, 1956, pp. 286–288, 298–299.

Mogul, K. Women in midlife: Decisions, rewards, and conflicts related to work and careers. *American Journal of Psychiatry*, 1979, *136*, 1139.

Nadelson, C., Polansky, D., & Mathews, M. Marital stress and symptom formation in midlife. *Psychiatric Opinion*, 1978, *15*, 29.

Neugarten, B. L. In I. Steinschein, (Reporter), The experience of separation–individuation . . . through the course of life: Maturity, senescence, and sociological implications (panel report), *Journal of the American Psychoanalytic Association*. 1973, *21*, 633.

Notman, M. Midlife concerns of women: Implications of the menopause. *American Journal of Psychiatry*, 1979, *136*, 1270.

Rich, A. *Snapshots of a daughter-in-law.* New York: W. W. Norton, 1967, pp. 11, 21–25, 47.

Rubin, L. B. *Women of a certain age: The midlife search for self.* New York: Harper & Row, 1979.

Rukeyser, M. *The gates.* New York: McGraw-Hill, 1976, p. 53.

Schaeffer, S. F. *Granite lady.* New York: Macmillan, 1974, pp. 40–41, 102.

Sexton, A. *Live or die.* New York: Houghton Mifflin, 1966, pp. 33, 62–65.

Sheehy, G. *Passages.* New York: E. P. Dutton, 1974.

Stewart, W. *A psychosocial study of the formation of the early adult life structure in women.* Unpublished doctoral dissertation, Columbia University, 1977.

10

Difficult Questions and Variations in Lifestyles

In the study of development, the same difficult questions arise over and over. Is development inevitable? Must everyone go through each stage to be normal? Who decides what is normal? Is development a cross-cultural phenomenon? What about the effects of education, social class, and money? In this chapter we will address such questions and relate them to concepts of adult development by discussing, as examples, such psychosocial phenomena as the effects of remaining single, divorcing, being widowed, and being homosexual.

MUST EVERYONE GO THROUGH THE SAME LIFE CYCLE?

Certain aspects of development, particularly those precipitated by genetically determined, maturational events, *are* inescapable and universal, such as readiness to walk and talk; perceptual and intellectual readiness to read and write; puberty; and the aging process in the adult body. Genetically determined events occur in essentially the same sequence in all human beings and, together with the environmental response to them, result in the forms, functions, and behavior that we call development.

Although less obvious, there are also inevitable and universal experiences underlying development in which psychological and environmental factors play significant or primary roles. Among those are the maternal response or the response of the mothering person(s) to the infant (Spitz, 1965); the parent–child interactions that determine identity in terms of sex and gender, as described by A. Freud (1963), Stoller (1968), and others; the adolescent interactions with parents, peers, and significant adults that lead to consolidation of character (Blos, 1968); and the adult relationships that determine the emergence of capacities for intimacy, parenting, and generativity.

Although our knowledge of developmental processes is rudimentary and we understand little of the relationship between the maturational and the environmental factors, every human being is shaped by the interactions between the two.

Is There "Normal" Variation in These Universal Experiences?

Within the basic developmental experiences common to all, there is profound and infinite variation, for each individual is, in fact, unique. Even between identical twins raised in the same family, differences in genetic predisposition, intelligence, patterns of growth, parental attitudes, acts of fate such as illness or accident result in distinct human beings.

Perhaps normal variation is best understood in terms of the concept of *developmental lines*, an idea formulated by Anna Freud (1963). By describing the manner and sequence in which various aspects of the personality unfold as a result of the interaction between biological and environmental factors, development is broken into manageable components for clarity and study. Examples are as follows: from suckling to rational eating; from wetting and soiling to bladder and bowel control; and the lines from the body to the toy and from play to work. Freud (1963) elaborates how the correspondence between developmental lines produces normal development and individuality:

> If we examine our notions of average normality in detail, we find that we expect a fairly close correspondence between growth on the individual developmental lines. In clinical terms this means that, to be a harmonious personality, a child who has reached a specific stage in the sequence toward emotional maturity (for example, object constancy), should have attained also corresponding levels in his growth toward bodily independence (such as bladder and bowel control, loosening of the tie between food and mother), in the lines toward companionship, constructive play, etc. We maintain this expectation of a norm even though reality presents us with many examples to the contrary. There are numerous children, undoubtedly, who show a very irregular pattern in their growth. They may stand high on some levels (such as maturity of emotional relations, bodily inde-

pendence, etc.) while lagging behind in others (such as play where they continue to cling to transitional objects, cuddly toys, or development of companionship where they persist in treating contemporaries as disturbances or inanimate objects) . . . .

We assume that with all normally endowed, organically undamaged children the lines of development indicated above are included in their constitution as inherent possibilities. What endowment lays down for them on the side of the id are, obviously, the maturational sequences in the development of libido and aggression . . . . For the rest, that is, for what singles out individual lines for special promotion in development, we have to look to accidental environmental influences. In the analysis of older children and the reconstructions from adult analysis we have found these forces embodied in the parents' personalities, their actions and ideals, the family atmosphere, the impact of the cultural setting as a whole . . . .

The disequilibrium between developmental lines . . . is not pathological as such, though it becomes a pathogenic agent where the imbalance is excessive. Moderate disharmony does no more than produce the many *variations of normality* with which we have to count. (pp. 262—264)

WHAT IS NORMAL? WHO DEFINES IT?

Obviously, there is no simple, all-inclusive definition of *normal*. We use the term here to refer to that mental activity and behavior which, based on current knowledge, falls within the broad range of predictable expectation, fulfills developmental potential, and is adaptive to the society in which it occurs. Of course there are many individuals, professional schools of thought, religions, and governments—all "defining" normal. So in that sense, society decides what is normal. And, we should add, not easily; witness the continual conflicts in Western society over rapidly changing ideas about marriage, divorce, abortion, the use of marijuana, homosexuality, and so on. The expectation that what is "normal" will change is built into our definition of development, because broad-based change is occurring continually in the environment and normal development is therefore subject to dynamic forces within the culture.

DO PEOPLE BYPASS STAGES OF DEVELOPMENT? WHAT HAPPENS WHEN THEY DO?

So far as we know, normal development is most likely to occur when the individual passes from phase to phase, engaging the developmental tasks in succession and to the fullest. This concept is valid for all major developmental theories, whether the stages have been proposed by S. Freud, Piaget, or Erikson. Each stage or task must be engaged to one degree or another, not necessarily successfully, and certainly not without conflict and turmoil. When stages are "bypassed"—which is not really possible—what results is either marked variation from the norms, or pathology.

Is Development a Cross-Cultural Phenomenon?

It has become clear in this century that development *is*, indeed, a cross-cultural phenomenon. This fact has been documented in large part by the work of such pioneer cultural anthropologists as Van Gennep, Benedict, Sapir, Mead, Bateson, and others, many of whom were familiar with if not influenced by psychoanalytic concepts of development. Van Gennep published his classic book, *Les rites de passage* in 1908, the same decade in which Freud published *The Interpretation of Dreams* (1900) and his ideas on development in infantile sexuality (1905). It was on that beginning that many who followed built what is known about development cross-cultural today.

Van Gennep firmly believed in the universality of development:

> The life of an individual in any society is a series of passages from one age to another and from one occupation to another . . . . We encounter a wide degree of general similarity among ceremonies of birth, childhood, social puberty, betrothal, marriage, pregnancy, fatherhood, initiation into religious societies, and funerals. In this respect, man's life resembles nature, from which neither the individual nor the society stands independent. The universe itself is governed by a periodicity which has repercussions on human life, with stages and transitions, movements forward, and periods of relative inactivity. (p. 3)

Although about 70 years separate the early work of Van Gennep and that of the contemporary anthropologist David Gutmann, they share the conviction that development is a cross-cultural phenomenon. Gutmann has sought to find the similarities in development among various cultures represented by five different groups: men in a midwestern American city (Kansas City) (1964); men in lowland (1966) and highland (1967) Mayan cultures of Mexico; men of the Navajo Indian tribe (Krohn & Gutmann, 1971); and an Islamic sect, the Druze of Israel (1974). He has verified with both cross-sectional and longitudinal data a basic developmental sequence in the lives of the men of all the societies he has examined (Gutmann, 1969, 1974, 1977), identifying three stages of adult development, each with characteristic attitudes toward the relationship between the world and the self.

The first stage, that of active mastery, encompasses roughly the years from 35 to 54. During that time the man has a productive orientation focused on actively dealing with and changing externals. In the second stage, which covers the decade from 54 to 64, passive mastery becomes the dominant mode; the man now views the world as a place where there are many things that he cannot change, and where his sources of pleasure and ways to meet his needs are most often not in his control but in the hands of forces or powers larger than himself. The final stage, beginning around age 65, Gutmann refers to as the stage of magical mastery; during this phase there is a move toward regression, receptivity, and magical solutions to problems.

Gutmann views culture as the modifier of these underlying developmental phases. The stages provide the psychological tendencies; the culture determines the options for acceptable expression of the tendencies. Although culture can amplify or retard these intrinsic orientations, it cannot abolish them. Gutmann may use different terms than Levinson, Darrow, Klein, Levinson, and McKee (1978), who also studied adult men, but they too share a belief that continuing development is a universal adult phenomenon.

Although it is clear that there are universal developmental experiences which transcend cultural barriers, it is equally apparent that societal effects on development lead to *cultural specificity*. Each culture, by manipulating developmental processes, produces adult personalities that are adaptive to that particular society and ensure the continuity and cohesiveness of the culture. Erikson (1950) gives an excellent illustration of this idea in his account of the child-rearing practices of the Sioux and Yurok Indians and the effects of those practices on each culture's traditions, relationships to the environment, and survival. For example, after describing the Sioux practices of unlimited breast feeding and strapping enraged babies up to their necks on cradleboard, he writes.

> What convergence can we see between the Sioux child's orality and the tribe's ethical ideals? We have mentioned generosity as an outstanding virtue required in Sioux life. A first impression suggests that the cultural demand for generosity received its early foundation from the privilege of en-

joying the nourishment and the reassurance emanating from unlimted breast feeding. The companion virtue of generosity was fortitude, in Indians a quality both more ferocious and more stoical than mere bravery. It included an easily aroused quantity of quickly available hunting and fighting spirit, the inclination to do sadistic harm to the enemy, and the ability to stand extreme hardship and pain under torture and self-torture. Did the necessity of supressing early biting wishes contribute to the tribe's always ready ferocity? If so, it cannot be without significance that the generous mothers themselves aroused a "hunter's ferocity" in their teething infants, encouraging an eventual transfer of the infant's provoked rage to ideal images of hunting, encircling, catching, killing and stealing.

We are not saying here that their treatment in babyhood *causes* a group of adults to have certain traits—as if you turned a few knobs in your child-training system and you fabricated this or that kind of tribal or national character. In fact, we are not discussing traits in the sense of irreversible aspects of character. We are speaking of goals and values and of the energy put at their disposal by child-training systems. Such values persist because the cultural ethos continues to consider them natural and does not admit of alternatives. They persist because they have become an essential part of an individual's sense of identity, which he must preserve as a core of sanity and efficiency. But values do not persist unless they work economically, psychologically, and spiritually; and I argue that to this end they must continue to be anchored, generation after generation, in early child training; while child training, to remain consistent, must be embedded in a system of continued economic and cultural synthesis. For it is the synthesis operating within a culture which increasingly tends to bring into close-knit thematic relationship and mutual amplification such matters as climate and anatomy, economy and psychology, society and child training. (pp. 137–138)

IS THE LIFE CYCLE AS WE HAVE DESCRIBED IT A CLASS PHENOMENON?

No, the major developmental themes within the human life cycle are not class phenomena. Universal themes in development cut across culture *and* class. But because of its effect on the immediate environment, class status does influence the form that development takes, a point substantiated by the work of Levinson and of Mayer (1978). As described in Chapter 3, Levinson and colleagues (1978) selected for their study a set of four occupations representing diverse sections of society that differed widely in type of work, origins, and the psychological and social conditions of their lives. They diversified their sample in terms of racial, ethnic, and religious origins: 15% were from poor urban or rural environments; 42% from working class or lower-middle class; 32% from comfortable middle class; and 10% from the wealthy class.

Until recently it was generally thought that only the affluent could afford to make career changes in midlife, but recent studies have shown that blue-collar workers struggle with the same developmental issues at midlife as their more affluent contemporaries. They experience need for change, renewal, and freedom of movement, and often they are willing to undergo considerable hardship to achieve their goals. Mayer (1978) describes the efforts of a group of 200 New York City policemen and firemen who became professional nurses. They attended classes three nights a week for 2½ years, and had to deal with the response of others to their changing from an extremely masculine career to one traditionally considered feminine. Their conscious reasons for making the change included wishes for security—guaranteed employment and supplemental retirement income—and for new work and challenge. Concerns about their bodies were also prominent; how would they tolerate physical danger and stress as they aged? As one of the policemen described the transition:

> It took a lot to sign up for this course, knowing the reactions we had to face back at the stationhouse. You have to have some guts to go ahead and say I'm going to change my whole conception of what I want to do, how I want to fulfill myself. . . . Like me, some of the guys are going around the clock. There are days you go to work, go to school, go home to sleep—and start again at 5:00 a.m. It's tough, and you're putting in a lot of time and effort. If a guy wants to change his job he has to have moxie. And if he doesn't, he's never going to do it. (pp. 207–208)

So there is a basic universal character to development which is experienced by all individuals, regardless of culture, class, or status. However, that universality stands in counterpoint to the great diversity which is also characteristic of human development. At no point in the life cycle is that diversity and variation more evident than at midlife, particularly in a culture in transition, like our own.

CHANGING SOCIAL PATTERNS

In this section we will attempt to relate the developmental framework to the social institutions of marriage and the family and to alternative life structures such as the single state, divorce, widowhood, and homosexuality—realities of life for an increasing number of individuals in contemporary society. Some of the changes taking place in our social institutions are described succinctly by Stevens-Long (1979).

> Since reaching a low point in the early 1950s, the divorce rate for first marriages has risen consistently over the past twenty-five years. In some ways, the 1950s were a period of reprieve from historical trends. A larger percentage of the population was married then than ever before or since, and people married younger in the 1950s than at any other time in recent history. The divorce rate which has peaked just after World War II, declined significantly, and the birth rate was extraordinarily high. Much of the American middle class moved to the spreading suburbs. Women left the work force and the rigors of collegiate and professional education. For middle America, these were the Eisenhower years—felt skirts, ducktails, and Sid Caesar.
>
> Since the 1950s, every one of these statistics has changed dramatically. Singlehood has regained some of its earlier popularity, the trip to the altar typically occurs later in the late 1970s than it did in the late 1950s, motherhood seems to have lost some of its luster, and the suburbs are strewn with the wreckage of lifelong monogamy gone awry. (pp. 142–143)

Our own attitude toward these changing social institutions and alternatives is one of inquiry. In developmental terms, one of the two major forces that shape development, the environment, is undergoing significant change. Our definition states that development is the *outcome* of the interaction between organism and environment. Thus the result will be changes in the developmental process. From those who choose to study the adult, those changes will require new attitudes, new questions, open-minded recognition of the limitations of our knowledge, and the evolution of new theories that can take into account the actuality of how people live and behave. As we did in Chapter 6 on the aging body, here we will present current data to use in formulating new developmental hypotheses.

The Family

A rapid evolution in the nature and structure of the family is occurring, with the emergence of new forms and variations on old ones. A somewhat conventional example is what Sussman and Burchinal (1962) call the *modified extended family*. An outgrowth of the closely knit, geographically bound, extended family common in Europe and in second- and some third-generation immigrant families in the United States, the modified extended family provides a mechanism for the maintenance of relationships among siblings and generations across differing local customs and great distances. In the United States today, many, possibly most, people live in modified extended families. Grandparents may live in the East while their children are scattered about the country. Grandchildren, with ready access to great mobility, may study or reside anywhere in the country, even in the world. Communication is maintained by telephone and visits made easier by air travel.

In the psychic lives of its members, the modified extended family is a real entity, affecting their thoughts and actions, providing sustenance, and contributing to identity. In our opinion, much has been lost by this evolution—the easy day-to-day contact, the warmth of frequent family gatherings, the ready support in times of crisis; but much has also been gained—freedom to evolve and think independently, to develop in ways less restricted by strong and sometimes rigid ethnic mores.

Kimmel (1974) lists other common family structures: (1) the one-parent family; (2) the extra-person family (housekeeper, aged parent, etc.); (3) the complex family, constructed after divorce and remarriage; and (4) homosexual families. Another significant variation in family living is the Israeli kibbutz, a structure that takes into account the needs of individuals at all phases of the life cycle (Talmon, 1961).

We have observed, as Kimmel has, functioning families of various structures in which children and parents manage to grow and develop. The relationship in such families have barely been studied in terms of their effects on development, and the task will be a challenging one:

> Thus, one "nuclear" family may consist of parts of two previous families living together during the week as a single family; but on weekends the members shift and visit their parents as if they were members of an extended family. If the relationships with the various sets of grandparents (at least six grandparents, perhaps eight or more) are included, the family structure becomes very complex, indeed. (Kimmel, 1974, p. 191)

Just as we conceptualize the individual as a developing organism changing throughout the life cycle, so do we view the family. Thinking about the family in such terms, as with the individual, tends to reduce stereotypic thinking, undermines the notion that the family is a monolithic, one-of-a-kind structure, and underscores the notion that family development occurs in a variety of forms, many of which may promote positive development.

Duvall (1971), Hill (1965), and Kimmel (1974) have described what may be called a cycle of development for the traditional family. Cycles for less traditional family structures remain to be described. In the traditional family the individual grows up in the family of origin; after leaving to marry and have children he enters the family of procreation, a phase that continues until the birth of the last child; the cycle continues, demarcated by the last child leaving home, and eventually widowhood.

The Single State

As of 1975 there were 43 million unmarried adults in the United States. In California alone there were 500,000 divorced, widowed, or never-married women who were heads of households (Edwards & Hoover, 1975). The increased numbers of single people may be related to the transformation of marriage in the Western world from primarily a unit of production of domestic goods to a source of emotional gratification and self-actualization (Melville, 1977). The belief that traditional marriage cannot meet the personal, social, and sensual needs of many individuals in contemporary society has led to the emergence of alternatives; hence the proposal of the single state as a developmental framework that can lead to fulfillment.

Edwards and Hoover (1975) point out the negative image of the single person in society and propose "a revolutionary change in attitude about the single life" (p. 12) because today

> we have a society with far different economic and social realities than have ever existed before, and there is no longer unanimity about the need for, or the ability of, marriage and childbearing to provide fulfillment for the individual or the society. (p. 19)

The women's movement, which has influenced our thinking, points out the advantages in the single life for women. Bernard (1972), for example, states that marriage is generally good for men because they expect care, comfort, and ordered domesticity, but may be hazardous for women, even make them emotionally ill, because their needs for self-identity are frequently not met in the home. That may explain why others report that single women are happier than single men and have lower rates of neuroses and depression than married women (Campbell, 1975).

Although descriptive and written from an advocate's viewpoint, the following advantages to being single proposed by Edward and Hoover (1975) contain suggestions of how the single state can promote the development of creativity, object ties, and healthy narcissism.

Privacy, being able to think and create without interruption in a peaceful atmosphere.

Time, having time to travel, cultivate talents, relax, entertain, be entertained.

Freedom, being able to choose, to make decisions, to form friendships, to use your time as you wish.

Opportunity, being able to extend borders of friendship, develop skills, move to new jobs and new places. (p. 39)

Separation, Divorce, and Remarriage

Although we have some understanding of the factors that cause divorce—for example, there are higher rates of divorce among children of divorced parents and between people whose marriages are childless or took place after a pregnancy had begun (Duvall, 1971)—little has been done to characterize the effect of divorce on adult-developmental tasks. In this brief discussion we can only hint at some of the areas that need to be explored.

Separation and divorce produce major changes in life structure, disrupting existing developmental lines, enhancing some while stifling others. For example, divorce might disrupt the developmental experiences of parenthood but enhance the development of intimacy by ending a sterile relationship and beginning an enriching one.

Nevertheless, such disruption requires the individual to engage a new subculture with its corresponding new norms, expectations, and rules of behavior. The major intrapsychic reorganization influences the person's identity, sense of self, ego ideal, and superego functioning and demands realignment of object ties and a restructuring of the ego to allow instinctual gratification in new settings with new individuals. All of that change takes place at a time when the adult may already be preoccupied with aging, time limitation, and other midlife developmental themes.

A 48-year-old father of four children, divorced three years, complained bitterly of his situation. He felt desperately lonely, unable to form a deep attachment to a woman. He was tired of casual sex and had come to realize that *many of the women he dated did not want to remarry.* They enjoyed the freedom of the single life; he did not. In addition, he felt that his children, who lived with him, desperately needed a mother. But how would any woman in her right mind choose to become the mother of four teen-agers? He felt a sense of urgency both for his children and for himself. Fifty was just around the corner.

Yet our patient seems to be the exception rather than the rule. There is no doubt that separation and divorce are major stresses. Individuals experiencing them have a higher incidence of admissions to mental hospitals than either married or widowed persons (Carter & Glick, 1970), but a large number of divorced persons do remarry, 75% within five years (Glick, 1949), and most second marriages are happier than first marriages and usually last until one of the partners dies (Hunt, 1966). Separation and divorce may result from unresolved individual or family psychopathology, but as evidenced by these statistics, they may be a mechanism for encouraging adult growth and development.

Widowhood

Widowhood is a major event affecting development in many adults, more women than men. In the 1972 United States Census (1973), there were 1.8 million widowed men and 9.6 million widowed women in the country, most of whom were over 65 (1.4 million men and 6.3 million women). The developmental tasks for these individuals are to mourn, to form new patterns in regard to work and activity, to become reinvolved with others in new ways, and possibly to remarry. Each of those steps requires the presence of an intact personality, continued physical health, and environmental receptivity—a difficult combination for older individuals to acquire. The degree of difficulty is suggested by the fact that the widowed have the highest death rate from accidental fire, accidental falls (women), suicide (men), and motor-vehicle accidents of any identified group (Carter & Glick, 1970).

The causes for such grim statistics may be related to the little-studied, poorly understood grief process in middle and old age. Goin and Burgoyne (1980) report "a conspiracy of silence between the bereaved and those who have not experienced the death of a loved one regarding the long-range effects of the loss" (p. 3). They discovered that in many healthy individuals the emotional attachment to a dead spouse, including subsequent recurrent episodes of painful grief, may remain *for many years*. Their finding has important implications for our understanding of development in midlife and old age. It leads us to hypothesize that the mourning process in later life may be qualitatively different than that in earlier stages of development, being more prolonged and more difficult to complete. This difference may be related to less flexibility in the aging, and often more rigid, ego, but also to the enormity of the loss. Not only the spouse is lost, but those aspects of living related to the spouse—identity, some peer and family relationships, sex, companionship, and so on.

Support systems often falter because those involved with the widowed need to deny the mourning process and its stimulation of their own thoughts about time limitation and death. One patient, describing her irritation at her father who was still mourning his wife's death after two years, expressed the wish that he'd "put on a happy face and get on with it." Most widowed individuals do indeed eventually "get on with it," for all major life changes, including the death of a spouse, provide the opportunity for growth as well as fixation.

> A 55-year-old woman came into treatment three years after the death of her husband. The mourning process was complicated by unrecognized and unresolved death wishes since in many ways her dictatorial spouse had stifled her development. Once free of that unconscious conflict, she attacked life with joyous abandon, traveling, experiencing increased sexual pleasure in new relationships, and pursuing a long-standing interest in music. Her developmental potential was realized in many new ways.

Homosexual Lifestyles

That considerable variation occurs within basic developmental patterns is a major tenet of our thinking. This premise appears to run counter to the tendency in human nature to stereotype members of unfamiliar social, ethnic, or racial groups and see them as undifferentiated from one another. That tendency may partially explain why those engaging in homosexual behavior have not been understood in the context of developmental complexity until fairly recently. Rather, *all* homosexuals were considered to be part of a monolithic, homogeneous group regarded as a "pathetic caricature of a fully sanctioning human being" (Bell & Weinberg, 1978).

Kinsey and his colleagues (Kinsey, Pomeroy, Martin, & Grebhard, 1948, 1953) were the first to challenge those stereotypes. Their work indicated that millions of Americans had engaged in homosexual activity, and they concluded that homosexual behavior was simply a natural variation of sexual expression. Their insight touched off considerable professional and scientific controversy because it was generally believed that adults who engaged in homosexual behavior were necessarily emotionally disturbed or less well adjusted than heterosexuals. The controversy continues to the present, debated by major professional organizations. Judd Marmor, a prominent psychoanalyst, urged the American Psychiatric Assocation to reexamine its views and definition of homosexuality:

> Surely the time has come for psychiatry to give up the archaic practice of classifying the millions of men and women who accept or prefer homosexual object choices as being, by virtue of that fact alone, mentally ill. The fact that their alternative lifestyle happens to be out of favor with current cultural conventions must not be a basis in itself for a diagnosis of psychopathology. (Marmor, 1973, p. 1209)

The outcome of the controversy as reflected in the American Psychiatric Association's *Diagnostic and Statistical Manual of Mental Disorders* (*DSM* III 1980) has been to remove homosexual behavior per se as an indication of a pathological sexual deviation. In the past (*DSM* II, 1968) the classification designated "Sexual Deviation" included all conditions in which the goal of the sexual behavior deviated from a defined norm of hetersexual coitus between adults and circumstances that would not be considered bizarre. Therefore homosexuality was included. In contrast, *DSM* III (1980) only includes as disorders those deviations from standard sexual behavior that involve gross impairment in the capacity for affectionate sexual activity between adult-human partners. Therefore homosexuality per se is not included as a sexual disorder. In their 10-year study commissioned by the National Institute of Mental Health, Bell and Weinberg (1978) continued the original Kinsey-Institute research on sexual behavior, and their data challenge the assumption that homosexually oriented people are very much alike, instead demonstrating considerable complexity and diversity of lifestyles within the homosexual world. They write:

> Our hope is that, at the very least, it will become increasingly clear to the reader that there is no such thing as *the* homosexual (or the heterosexual for that matter) and that statements of any kind which are made about human beings on the basis of their sexual orientation must always be highly qualified . . . .As long as homosexual men and women, as well as other groups of people who are simply seen as "different" from the majority of American citizens, continue to be viewed through stereotypical thinking, our society will pay the price inevitably exacted by fear and ignorance. We hope that our present work will help to diminish the forces of interpersonal alienation and enable people to become increasingly reconciled to themselves as well as to others. (pp. 23–25)

Kinsey and colleagues (1948) first reported that nearly half of American males fell somewhere between exclusively heterosexual and exclusively homosexual. Bell and Weinberg (1978) similarly found a wide spectrum of experience on the homosexual–heterosexual continuum as reflected in mixed homo-heterosexual feelings, behaviors, dreams, and fantasies. Homosexual diversity was also evident in levels of sexual activity, cruising patterns, variation in sexual techniques, levels of sexual interest, and the incidence of sexual problems.

Most relevant for our study of adult development are their data about the nature of sexual partnerships among homosexual men and women, which call into question some commonly held assumptions:

> One of the most predominant images of the homosexual man is that he is highly "promiscuous," unable to integrate his emotional and sexual needs, incapable of maintaining a longstanding sexual partnership, and doomed to an eternally hopeless quest for the ideal relationship. His proclivity for "impersonal, expedient, and fleeting encounters" (Humphreys, 1971) is frequently juxtaposed with the lesbian's supposed interest in a permanent "marriage" to another woman and her much greater preoccupation with sexual fidelity. (p. 81)

However, rather than inferior imitations of heterosexual premarital or marital involvements, the relatively steady relationships that homosexual men or women form with their partners are, according to Bell and Weinberg's research, very meaningful in their lives.

> From our respondents' descriptions, these affairs are apt to involve an emotional exchange and commitment similar to the kinds that heterosexuals experience, and most of the homosexual respondents thought they and their partners had benefited personally from their involvement and were at least somewhat unhappy when it was over. The fact that they generally went on to a subsequent affair with another partner seems to suggest a parallel with heterosexuals' remarriage after divorce rather than any particular emotional immaturity or maladjustment. In any case, most of our homosexual respondents spoke of these special relationships in positive terms and clearly were not content to limit their sexual contacts to impersonal sex. (p. 102)

Another important related finding contradicted the commonly held stereotype that homosexual men and women are sex-ridden individuals who think constantly of sexual matters or consider sex the most important part of their lives. The data demonstrated a diversity of sexual interest among the respondents, clearly indicating that for a significant number of homosexuals, sex was not a particularly dominant concern.

A Typology of Homosexual Men

In our opinion, the most meaningful result to emerge from Bell and Weinberg's research was the demonstration of definite, descriptive subgroups indicating varying degrees of maturity along developmental lines. Included were individuals who are able to work, love, and play successfully; intermediates who do so to varying degrees; and finally a group of homosexual men and women who are lonely, depressed, and basically socially dysfunctional.

Using a factor-analysis statistical approach, Bell and Weinberg assigned their respondents to five groups: (1) close coupled, (2) open coupled, (3) functional, (4) dysfunctional, and (5) asexual.

Close Coupled. Sixty-seven men were assigned to this group. The criterion for being included was involvement in a quasi-marriage with a male partner. Close-coupled homosexuals had fewer sexual problems and fewer partners, and cruised less than the typical male respondent. In addition, individuals in this group had fewer difficulties finding an appropriate partner and maintaining affection for him as well as less regret about their homosexuality, and they were more sexually active than the typical respondent.

Open Coupled. The 120 men assigned to this group were involved in "marital" relationships also, but their standard scores were high on one or more of the following variables: number of sexual partners, number of sexual problems, and amount of cruising. Unlike the close-coupled males, these men's special relationships had not reduced their sexual problems or their interest in a variety of sexual contacts. The open coupled group tended to be more exclusively homosexual, to engage in a wider variety of sexual techniques, and to have more regret about their homosexuality. Their partner's failure to respond to their sexual requests was reported as their most prevalent sexual problem.

Functional. One-hundred-two men were assigned to this subgroup. These single individuals had high standard scores in regard to number of sexual partners and level of sexual activity and low ones on regret over their homosexuality. They were more overtly homosexual, had a higher level of sexual interest, more extensive sexual repertoires, and a sense of ease and acceptance of their homosexuality.

Dysfunctional. By definition, none of the 86 men in this group was coupled. They had a high number of partners, many sexual problems, and much regret about their homosexuality. Their sexual problems were related to concerns about sexual adequacy, difficulties in reaching orgasm, finding appropriate sexual partners, and maintaining affection for the partners they did find.

Asexual. One-hundred-ten men were considered by the research group to be relatively asexual on the basis of their standard scores. None of them was in a coupled relationship. They scored low on level of sexual activity, number of partners, and amount of cruising. These men reported much lower levels of sexual interest, less extensive sexual repertoires, and significant regret about their homosexuality.

A Typology of Homosexual Women

In analyzing the data from their female respondents, Bell and Weinberg used the same methods they had used in studying homosexual males. They had no particular interest in creating comparable or even the same number of male and female groups. However, the data on homosexual women sorted into an identical number of groups, that is, five, that could be described in the same terms, that is, close coupled, open coupled, and so on, and were directly comparable in most respects. One significant difference was the greater number of women designated as close coupled.

Developmental Implications

Data on various homosexual adaptations serve to illustrate the points made earlier in this chapter about adult-developmental diversity and variation. Moreover, the data demonstrate the *complexity* of the developmental processes and the interdigitation of developmental lines by indicating that sexual development does not in and of itself preclude or determine development along other lines such as career, friendships, creativity, and so on. Variations in lifestyle provide an opportunity for research and study of developmental issues, serving almost as "natural experiments" in themselves. However, since variations such as the homosexualities run counter to the culture, there are secondary spin-offs which make study difficult and generalizations hard to arrive at.

Now that homosexuality is being discussed and studied somewhat more openly in our culture, more and more examples of talented, successful homosexuals are appearing. Both developmental diversity and successful development along a number of lines are well illustrated in Morgan's (1980) study of the novelist Somerset Maugham's life. Maugham was bisexual, and his homosexuality was the great secret of his life. Morgan described the richness and complexities of Maugham's personality and the different roles he played at different stages of his life. Maugham was an alienated child, a medical student, a bohemian in Paris, a successful playwright, a spy in Russia, a promiscuous homosexual, a cuckolded husband, a World-War-II propagandist, the most widely read novelist of his time, and a living legend who tried to disinherit his daughter and adopt his secretary in his senility.

It must be recognized, however, that a successful variation in lifestyle, such as Maugham's, does not negate the significance of the universal nature of the *conflicts* and *tasks* associated with all stages of development and with all developmental outcomes. What is common to all human beings is the need to engage their homosexual impulses. For most people the result of the conflict is a sublimation of homosexual drives and an increasing differentiation of heterosexual ones; for homosexuals the opposite tends to occur. Both engage the same developmental issues and tasks; only the outcomes are different.

In recognizing the developmental variation possible for human beings, it becomes clear that all adults are best understood as whole human beings, in all their complexities, not just in terms of one aspect of their behavior.

References

Bell, A., & Weinberg, M. *Homosexualities: A study of diversity among men and women.* New York: (Touchstone) Simon & Schuster, 1978.

Bernard, J. *The future of marriage.* New York: World Publishing Corp., 1972.

Blos, P. Character formation in adolescence. *Psychoanalytic Study of the Child,* 1968, 23, 245.

Campbell, A. The American way of mating: Marriage, sex, children. *Psychology Today,* May, 1975, p. 39.

Carter, H., & Glick, P. C. *Marriage and divorce: A social and economic study.* Cambridge: Harvard University Press, 1970.

Diagnostic and statistic manual of mental disorders II. Washington, D.C.: American Psychiatric Association, 1968.

Diagnostic and statistical manual of mental disorders III. Washington: American Psychiatric Association, 1980.

Duvall, E. M. *Family development* (4th ed.). Philadelphia: J. B. Lippincott, 1971.

Edwards, M., & Hoover, E. *The challenge of being single.* New York: Signet Books, 1975.

Erikson, E. H. *Childhood and society.* New York: W. W. Norton, 1950.

Freud, A. The concept of developmental lines. *Psychoanalytic Study of the Child*, 1963, *18*, 245.

Freud, S. Standard edition, Vols. 4 and 5. London: Hogarth Press, 1900.

Freud, S. *Three essays on the theory of sexuality*. Standard edition, 7:125. London: Hogarth Press, 1905.

Galenson, E., & Roiphe, H. The impact of early sexual discovery on mood, defense organization, and symbolization. *Psychoanalytic Study of the Child*, 1971, *26*,195.

Glick, P. C. First marriages and remarriages. *American Sociological Review*, 1949, *14*, 726.

Goin, M. K., & Burgoyne, R. W. *Psychology of the widow and widower*. Unpublished manuscript, 1980.

Gutmann, D. L. An exploration of ego configurations in middle and later life. In B. L. Neugartern (Ed.), *Personality in middle and later life*. New York: Atherton Press, 1964, pp. 114–148.

Gutmann, D. L. Mayan aging: A comparative TAT study. *Psychiatry*, 1966, *29*, 246.

Gutmann, D. L. Aging among the highland Maya: A comparative study. *Journal of Personal and Social Psychology*, 1967, *1*, 28.

Gutmann, D. L. The country of old men: Cultural studies in the psychology of later life. *Occasional papers in gerontology* (No. 5). Ann Arbor: Institute of Gerontology, University of Michigan, 1969, pp. 1–37.

Gutmann, D. L. Alternatives to disengagement: The old men of the highland Druze. In R. A. Levine (Ed.), *Culture and personality*. Chicago: Aldine, 1974, pp. 232–245.

Gutmann, D. L. The Cross-cultural perspective: Notes toward a comparative psychology of aging. In J. E. Birren & K. W. Schaie (Eds.), *Handbook of the psychology of aging*. New York: Van Nostrand Reinhold, 1977, pp. 302–326.

Hill, R. Decision making and the family life cycle. In E. Shanas & G. Streib (Eds.), *Social structure and the family: Generational reactions*. Englewood Cliffs, N.J.: Prentice-Hall, 1965, pp. 113–139.

Humphreys, R. A. New styles in homosexual manliness. *Transaction*, March–April, 1971, p. 30.

Hunt, M. M. *The world of the formerly married*. New York: McGraw-Hill, 1966.

Kimmel, D. C. *Adulthood and aging*. New York: Wiley, 1974.

Kinsey, A. C., Pomeroy, W. B., Martin, C. E., & Gebhard, P. H. *Sexual behavior in the human male*. Philadelphia: W. B. Saunders, 1948.

Kinsey, A. C., Pomeroy, W. B., Martin, C. E., & Gebhard, P. H. *Sexual behavior in the human female*. Philadelphia: W. B. Saunders, 1953.

Krohn, A., & Gutmann, D. L. Changes in mastery style with age: A study of Navajo dreams. *Psychiatry*, 1971, *34*, 289.

Levinson, D. J., Darrow, C. N., Klein, E. B., Levinson, M. H., & McKee, B. *The seasons of a man's life*. New York: Alfred A. Knopf, 1978.

Marmor, J. Homosexuality and cultural value systems. *American Journal of Psychiatry*, 1973, *130*, 1209.

Mayer, N. *The male mid-life crisis: Fresh starts after forty*. New York: Doubleday, 1978.

Melville, K. *Marriage and family today*. New York: Random House, 1977.

Morgan, T. *Maugham*. New York: Simon & Schuster, 1980.

Spitz, R. *The first year of life*. New York: International Universities Press, 1965.

Stevens-Long, J. *Adult life*. Palo Alto, Calif.: Mayfield, 1979.

Stoller, R. J. *Sex and gender*. New York: Science House, 1968.

Sussman, M. B., & Burchinal, L. Kin family network: Unheralded structure in current conceptualizations of family functioning. *Marriage and Family Living*, 1962, *24*, 231.

Talmon, Y. Aging in Israel, a planned society. *American Journal of Sociology*, 1961, *67*, 284.

United States Bureau of the Census. *Some demographic aspects of aging in the United States.*
    Current Population Reports, Series P-23, No. 32. Washington, D.C.: United States
    Government Printing Office, 1973.
Van Gennep, A. *The rites of passage.* Chicago: University of Chicago Press, 1960. (Origi-
    nally published, 1908.)

III

APPLICATIONS

11

The Adult-Developmental Diagnosis

Developmental concepts alter the diagnostic process with adult patients because they influence the therapist's attitude about the patient and his problems, the collection and recording of data, and the diagnosis and treatment formulations. Since our focus and aim are specific, we will not comment on many accepted aspects of standard diagnostic technique and suggest that the interested reader acquaint himself with such basic texts as *The American Handbook of Psychiatry* (Stevenson, 1965) or *The Technique of Psychotherapy* (Wolberg, 1967) for such purposes. Furthermore, there is no single correct way to do a diagnosis evaluation and our method should be accepted as one approach that can be adapted by each therapist to his or her individual style.

PURPOSE

The purpose of doing an adult, developmental, diagnostic evaluation is to collect relevant data about a patient that will lead to a clear understanding of the normal and deviant developmental factors from childhood and adulthood which underlie the patient's healthy growth and symptomatology. This developmental construction, coupled with a psychodynamic understanding of the patient's *intrapsychic conflicts* and a knowledge of his physical state and environmental interactions, brings together the information required to make a comprehensive diagnosis and formulate a practical treatment plan.

It is important to note that we are describing diagnostic procedures for the *individual*, who remains, for us, the basic unit of observation, study, and intervention. Other valid orientations such as family or systems theory require different diagnostic techniques, which can be complementary to rather than competitive with an individual approach. But the individual does not live in isolation. Therefore individual diagnostic procedures must take into account and explore the network of *interdependent* relationships with other adults and children who influence all aspects of adult development.

OUTLINE OF THE DIAGNOSTIC EVALUATION

An outline of the adult, developmental, diagnostic evaluation is as follows:

    I. History
        A. Identifying information
        B. Chief complaint(s)
        C. History of the present illness
        D. Developmental history
        E. Family history
   II. Additional Procedures
        A. Medical evaluation
        B. Psychological testing
  III. Diagnostic Impression
   IV. Treatment Plan
    V. Summary Conference

Let us turn our attention to the details of the evaluation.

Diagnostic Interviews

The initial interviews with the nonpsychotic adult are usually free flowing, the content determined largely by the patient. In subsequent interviews the therapist elaborates the chief complaints by asking questions that fill in gaps in knowledge. Enough information should be obtained so that in recording the history the therapist can describe each symptom clearly, give a chronological picture of its development, and list those environmental and intrapsychic factors that influence its course.

Since the basic purpose of the evaluation is to identify the factors that underlie symptoms, not merely describe the symptoms themselves, the diagnostician should immediately begin to look for and evaluate both infantile and adult developmental themes. Among adult factors to be studied are attitudes about the body; feelings about important interpersonal relationships such as spouse, children, parents, and friends; and attitudes toward such basic issues as time and death or work and play. For example, the diagnostician must assess the patient's attitude toward his body. He could begin by noting what the patient says about his body and what he does with it. Manner of dress, weight level, carriage and bearing, alterations such as dyed hair or cosmetic surgery, and physical impairments are all clues that help the diagnostician determine how the patient is reacting to physical aging.

Frequently the chief complaint itself is a direct expression of an adult-developmental theme. Examples: "I'm depressed because my children are leaving home." "I need to make more money but I'm afraid to change my job. I know it's all in my head. Can you help me?"

In many instances attitudes toward the therapist and treatment are strongly colored from the first contact on by adult-developmental issues. For instance, the relative ages of the therapist and patient as perceived by the patient may influence the course of the interviews. Older patients may treat a younger therapist as a son or daughter in an attempt to control the interaction while a patient of the opposite sex but same age may act seductively or withhold sexual material out of unrecognized sexual attraction or embarrassment.

The Developmental History

Detailed developmental histories are routinely done in the evaluation of children but often neglected in the evaluation of adults. This practice persists because of the widely held notion that developmental processes play a minor role in the adult, and because of the absence until recently of an adult-developmental theory from which to derive necessary diagnostic tools, such as a developmental-history outline, for the adult. It is our belief that a developmental history that describes the entire life experience of the patient—from conception to the present—should be taken from each adult patient. Later in this chapter we present an outline for a developmental history of the life cycle and a detailed case history illustrating its use.

As with the history of the present illness, this information is obtained by first asking the patient to describe in his own manner and sequence those developmental experiences most important to him; followed by questions from the examiner about areas of child and adult development that require further elaboration. The idea is not to monotonously and compulsively elicit details but to gain as clear a perspective as possible of major trends and experiences. Above all, the goal is to make the patient's life *understandable*.

Family History

The family history usually consists of a study of the parents, siblings, and relatives during the formative childhood years. Such information is basic and necessary and should be complemented by the *addition* of an account of experience with family members during the adult years as well. Many aspects of the patient's interaction with his family can be covered in both the developmental and family history and should include vignettes about interactions at such critical junctures as separations, marriages, births, deaths, and so on.

In midlife, themes such as caring for aging parents; as well as grandparent–grandchildren, grown child–parent, and spouse–parent relationships should be explored. The basic idea is to trace the *adult course* of the relationship between grown child and parent since their interaction continues to have a significant effect upon development.

> One 43-year-old man was very surprised by the intensity of emotion that welled up in him when asked about the death of his mother, which had occurred when he was 39. The therapist's questions about the circumstances of her death, the funeral, its effect on the patient's life, and so on led to a series of associations from both childhood and adulthood which greatly impressed upon the prospective patient the power of the diagnostic-therapeutic process and increased his desire for treatment.

Even patients in their fifties, sixties, and seventies will focus on parents—usually dead by this point—if the therapist is sensitive enough to inquire and listen. It is our impression that feelings about parents remain dynamically charged in elderly patients and—if not dismissed by the therapist as boring reminiscenses of the distant past—can lead to meaningful insight and therapeutic progress. Feelings about siblings, alive or dead, are of the same order of importance as those about parents, and should be explored in the same way.

Underlying this whole approach to the family history is the idea that the family of childhood has not vanished from the patient's life. It remains alive and potent, in altered form, in the intrapsychic life of the adult. Interactions with family, real and/or intrapsychic, continue to have a significant effect on development throughout the second half of the life cycle.

Diagnosis and Treatment Formulations

In order to make a comprehensive diagnostic statement, we suggest that the diagnostic formulation be broken down into three distinct parts: descriptive, dynamic, and developmental.

The *descriptive formulation* places the patient's symptoms into generally agreed-upon categories such as those presented in the *Diagnostic and Statistical Manual of Mental Disorders* of the American Psychiatric Association (1980). In our opinion, any diagnosis that is largely descriptive, although useful for communicative purposes, is inadequate by itself to convey a meaningful portrait of the patient's healthy and deviant development. However, it should be used in combination with the other two approaches.

The *dynamic formulation*, which explains the patient's problems and symptoms in terms of intrapsychic conflict, uses Freud's topographical formulation (conscious and unconscious) and structural theory (id, ego, and superego) to describe the conflicting impulses and defenses which underlie symptoms.

The *developmental formulation* traces the relationship between symptoms and conflicts and the major developmental occurrences at each phase of the life cycle that lead to their formation. Here is encapsulated a brief, cogent outline of the developmental experiences that give *uniqueness* to this particular individual.

Many diagnosticians include the developmental formulation as part of a broader dynamic formulation, feeling that developmental factors are only one category of several which produce the dysfunction observed. We have no basic quarrel with such a formulation but do feel that singling out the developmental factors involved in symptom formation leads to a clearer understanding of their emergence and meaning and to a greater appreciation of their interference with the forward thrust of development.

Treatment recommendations are not random but follow closely from the diagnostic conclusions arrived at following a thorough evaluation. The addition of adult-developmental concepts ensures greater flexibility and latitude in treatment planning. For example, older patients in their fifties or sixties and beyond are considered to be still evolving; thus they are potentially suitable for dynamic forms of treatment, including intensive psychotherapy and psychoanalysis. Their current developmental problems, which are not understood only as recapitulations of a distant past or preludes to death, take on a new significance and dignity in the mind of the therapist, which can lead to an enriched relationship between therapist and patient. Since the furthering of the developmental process is the basic goal of treatment, equal importance is given to intrapsychic factors, physical problems, and realistic environmental issues such as financial planning for retirement. Support, reassurance, chemotherapy, and dynamic psychotherapeutic techniques are used in concert with each other as indicated.

RECORDING THE EVALUATION

What follows is a suggested schema for recording the evaluation. What makes this schema unique is the inclusion of a detailed developmental history for the adult. In constructing it we have abstracted the major developmental themes of adulthood, thus providing the diagnostician with an organized outline of areas of development to be explored. Although for emphasis we make an arbitrary distinction between the development-history outline for childhood and for adulthood, both are part of a unified statement of the patient's life experience from birth through the present.

Identifying Information

a. Patient's full name, age, occupation, description
b. Spouse or partner's full name, age, occupation, description
c. Children—in chronological order—full name, age, major life activity, description
d. Others living in the home—name, age, major life activity, description, reason for presence in the home

The identifying information provides a basic grid on which to build a comprehensive picture of the patient.

Referral Source

By whom and for what reason was the patient referred? Knowledge of the manner in which the patient came for treatment—self-referred vs. referral by physician or spouse—provides a method for assessing motivation and serves as a reminder to the diagnostician to thank and send results of the evaluation to the referral source.

Chief Complaint(s)

a. In the patient's words
b. In the words of other family members, when different or relevant
c. In the words of the referral source, such as a physician

It is not unusual for the chief complaint to vary considerably, reflecting different facets of the problem or indicating the varying effects of the problem upon different family members or the community. Examples: Patient: "I'm depressed." Wife: "My husband has lost interest in me sexually. He's also avoiding the older children." Family physician: "George was a real steady guy until a year ago when he began complaining about vague GI pains. I couldn't find anything."

History of the Present Illness

Each symptom should be presented separately and described (1) clearly and concisely, (2) chronologically (when it started, how it changed over time, its present state), and (3) in terms of what, if anything, influences the symptom, makes it better or worse.

Developmental History

In taking a developmental history we are learning about the past in order to relate it to the person's present and future. An in-depth, dynamic understanding of symptoms and behavior is impossible without a knowledge of those factors in the life experience of this particular individual that cause him to think and act the way he does.

What follows is a suggested outline for a *developmental history of the life cycle* that covers the individual's life from birth to the chronological present and includes attitudes about the future. The outline for the childhood years is typical and a reworking of an outline by Kolansky and Stennis (1964). The adult-developmental outline is our own formulation—a distillation of the major adult-developmental themes as we now understand them.

Childhood

Adults will not have actual memories of infancy or early childhood, but they will have surprising amounts of secondhand information received from parents or relatives. Despite the inevitable inaccuracies and distortions involved, it is possible to establish many basic facts about the early-childhood years; for example, the presence or absence of mother, illnesses, operations, thumb sucking, bed wetting, and so on. Of equal importance is the emergence of the patient's *intrapsychic* image of his childhood relationships and experiences. The following areas should be explored with the patient.

Pregnancy
Planned or unplanned
Parental sex preference
Normal or problem pregnancy—medication
Bleeding, illness, weight gain, etc.
Maternal psychological health—mood, living situations, relationship to father
Full term or premature

Labor and delivery
Spontaneous or induced
Length of labor
Complications
Vertex or breech presentation
Natural or Caesarean birth
Birth weight
Involvement of the father

First year of life (oral phase)
Selection of name
Feeding patterns, breast or bottle fed. Maternal involvement and attitudes

Circumcision, bris
Quality and quantity of mothering, fathering
Sleep–wake patterns
Sleeping arrangements
Temperament
Developmental milestones—first sitting, walking, etc.
Smile response, stranger anxiety
Thumb sucking, use of pacifier
Weaning
Separation–individuation process—autistic and symbiotic phases
Parents' relationship with each other—effect on infant
Illness and operations—throughout childhood
Major parental absences, illnesses, or death
Moves—throughout childhood

Ages 1–3 (anal phase)
Language development—first appearance of single words, sentences
Motor development—locomotion, fine- and gross-motor coordination
Separation–individuation process-maternal availability, independence vs. clinging behavior, ability to tolerate brief separations, etc., establishment of object constancy
Establishment of core gender identity
Toilet training—when begun, when and how accomplished, by whom, family attitudes about bowel and bladder functioning
Enuresis, encopresis
Aggressiveness, negativism—"terrible twos"
Parental attitudes toward limits, controls, punishments

Ages 3–6 (oepidal phase)
Sexual curiosity, exploration, masturbation
Dreams, nightmares
Phobias
Attitudes toward parent of the same sex, opposite sex
Family nudity, showering, bathing with children
Parental attitudes toward sexual questions, sexual play
Parental seductiveness, punitiveness
Actual seductions, primal scene, etc.

Early school experiences—ability to separate, relate to others, learn

Continued motor and perceptual development—riding tricycle, holding crayons, reading readiness, etc.

Ages 7–11 (latency)

School—academic progress vs. learning problems; capacity to relate to teachers, peers

Conscience formation

Involvement with peers—acceptance vs. isolation

Evidence of latency—age play; organized, group games

Development of hobbies, skills, sports, etc.

Sexual identification

Involvement with parents, particularly of the same sex

Adolescence

Pubertal development—when occurred, understanding of the experience, parental attitudes

Menstration/ejaculation—first experiences and attitudes

Masturbation

Attitudes about the development of the body

Mood swings, inconsistent behavior

Regressions

Relationship to parents

Relationship to peers

Heterosexual orientation and experience, dating, falling in love, intercourse

Homosexual orientation and experience

School accomplishments

Career planning, work experience

Hobbies and interests

Capacity for abstract thinking

Religious attitudes—throughout childhood

Adulthood

The adult developmental history will be presented in two ways: first chronologically in terms of adult developmental stages, thus providing continuity with the childhood developmental history, secondly in terms of adult developmental lines, thus singling out major adult-developmental themes and presenting them more comprehensively. When the developmental history is being taken from a patient the diagnostician will actually be *conceptualizing* the material in both ways.

Erikson (1963) divided adulthood into three phases—early, middle, and late. Levinson, Darrow, Klein, Levinson, and McKee (1978), building on Erikson's pioneer work, organized the life cycle into overlapping spans of 20 to 25 years as follows:

Preadulthood: Ages 0–22
Early adulthood: Ages 17–45
Middle adulthood: Ages 40–65
Late adulthood: Ages 60–85
Late, late adulthood: Age 80 and beyond

Further elaborating on these subdivisions, focusing partially on intrapsychic complexity, we have decided, with Erikson, to divide adulthood into early, middle, and late. The assignment of chronological ages to these stages is approximate, flexible, and meant to be descriptive, facilitating organized thinking. We are more interested in presenting the reader with the dynamic adult developmental tasks that roughly occur within these arbitrary chronological demarcations than with the phases themselves.

Early adulthood (ages 20–40)
Attitudes about and use of the body
Beginning sense of personal history, of time limitation
Attitudes about and experiences with death
Sexual experience—heterosexual, homosexual
Capacity for intimacy
Spouse-child-self relationships
Children—desire for, relationship with
Parents—psychological separation from, relationship with
Role of friendships
Choosing and establishing a career, creativity
Role as a mentee
Finances—use of money to further development
Expressions and forms of adult play

Conceptualization of role in society
Religious attitudes and activities

Middle adulthood (ages 40–60)
The middle-aged body—effects of physical change, illness, altered
    body image, etc.
Menopause, male climacteric
Attitudes toward time
Illness and death of contemporaries, parents
Reaction to parental death
Middle-age sexual drive, activity, intimacy
Relationship to spouse, partner
Relationship to adult children, grandchildren
Interaction with aging parents
Friendship—Long standing, new partial replacements for loss of
    children
"Resonance" with friends of all ages
Position of work, of play
Role as a mentor
Creativity
Attitudes toward money—for present, retirement, family, society
Society—attitude toward, position in, acceptance of change

Late adulthood (ages 60 and beyond)
Maintenance of body integrity—exercise, care, etc.
Reaction to physical infirmity, permanent impairment
Attitudes toward personal death
Integrity vs. despair (Erikson)
Reaction to death of spouse, friends
Attitudes toward, preoccupation with recent and distant past vs.
    present and future
Ability to form new ties
Reversal of roles with children, grandchildren
Companionship vs. isolation and loneliness
Role of sexual activity
Retirement—use of time, continuance of meaningful activity, work
    and play
Financial planning—attitudes toward self-care, surviving family
    members, society

Adult Developmental Lines

In attempting to assess a particular aspect of adult development, the concept of developmental lines (Freud, 1965) is particularly useful. The following outlines of some of the major themes in adult development are means to help the diagnostician organize his thoughts about his adult patient and provide a framework from which to phrase appropriate diagnostic questions and formulate diagnosis and treatment.

Intimacy, Love, and Sex

(Late teens and early 20s)
> Finding appropriate heterosexual partners
> Desire for sexual and nonsexual closeness
> Emergence of capacity for heterosexual caring, tenderness
> Ability to use the body comfortably as a sexual instrument
> Continued resolution of homosexual trends

(20s and 30s)
> Capacity to invest in one person—based on ability to trust enough, and to expose and tolerate imperfections in the self and the partner
> Continued broadening of sexual exploration and activity
> Wish for children as an expression of love, union, and sexuality
> Ability to share children with partners

(40s–50s)
> Increased recognition of the value of long-standing relationships
> Redefinition of relationships to partner as children grow and leave
> Ability to care for partner in face of illness, aging, physical retrogression
> Capacity to share new activities, interests, and people
> Continuation of active sex life
> Acceptance of diminished intensity of sexual drive
> Acceptance of loss of procreative ability in women

(60s–70s)
> Capacity to tolerate loss, death of partner, friends
> Ability to form new sustaining ties with friends, children, grandchildren
> Continuation of active sex life, including masturbation in absence of a partner

The Body

(Late teens and early 20s)

Attitudes toward the body—casual acceptance, concerns, invincibility vs. vulnerability, etc.

Development of physical abilities, prowess

Care of the body—exercise, weight control, etc., vs. neglect

(30s–40s)

Growing awareness of physical limitations

Attitudes toward baldness, grey hair, wrinkles, changes in vision, diminished strength, etc.

Normal mourning for the body of youth

Emergence of new body image

Acceptance and integration of physical limitations and enjoyment of body in new ways

Continued care or neglect

(50s–60s)

Reactions to experience of physical decline

Reactions to physical impairment—hearing or vision loss, heart attacks, cancer, etc.

Ability to compensate for diminished physical energy—altering schedule, diet, sleep patterns, etc.

Care of the body—regular exercise, physical checkups, appropriate diet, vs. neglect

(70s)

Ability to remain active and outgoing in the face of frequent physical infirmity

Acceptance of permanent physical impairment—hearing, vision, etc.

Continued exercise and care of the body vs. neglect in the face of limited physical abilities

Time and Death

(Late teens and 20s)

Beginning awareness of a personal history

Increased cognizance and differentiation of personal past, present, and future

Sense of future time as almost unlimited

Little preoccupation with time or death

(30s–40s)

Increased awareness of personal time limitation

Personal experiences with death of parents, contemporaries

Developmental effects of midlife preoccupation with time and death, progressive and/or regressive—the midlife crisis

(50s–60s)

Acceptance of the preciousness of time, leading to increased interest in the quality of experience

Effect of personal vulnerability, illness, aging on thoughts of time and death

Effect of death of loved ones

Continued interest in present and future vs. dwelling on the past

(70s)

Integrity vs. despair (Erikson)

Preparation for personal death

Placing of one's life cycle in the span of family, national, and human history

Relationship to Children

(Late teens and 20s)

Desire for—as a confirmation of masculinity or femininity

Ability to care for, nurture

Capacity to subordinate personal needs to parenting functions

Integrating of parenting role with work identity, other interests, etc.

(30s–40s)

Willingness to love and set limits

Reworking of attitudes and conflicts over aggression in relation to limit setting

Tendency to punitive, envious overrestrictiveness vs. seductive encouragement of premature sexuality

Envy of adolescent's abundant future vs. adult's time limitation

Effect (on middle-age development) of interaction with adolescent children

Effect of relationship with growing children on marriage

Mourning for loss of role as parent of young children

Acceptance and encouragement of separation and independence in children

Mourning for loss of children

(50s–60s)

> Facilitation of adult children's development—emotionally, financially
>
> Establishment of mature friendships with grown children
>
> Acceptance of new sexual/life partners of grown children
>
> Acceptance of one's position in the older generation—grandparenthood
>
> Relationship to grandchildren

(70s)

> Continued facilitation of grown children's and grandchildren's development
>
> Acceptance of reversal of roles—help, support from middle-aged children

Relationship to Parents

(Late teens and 20s)

> Ability to psychologically and physically separate
>
> Dependency vs. independence in relation to continued financial and emotional support
>
> Forging of a separate identity
>
> Recognition and acceptance of parental limitations and imperfections
>
> Ability to establish an adult-to-adult relationship

(30s–40s)

> Evolution of adult-to-adult relationships, friendships
>
> Reaction to the aging process in parents
>
> Facilitation of parent's role as a grandparent
>
> Mourning, integration of parent's death

(50s and beyond)

> Acceptance of reversal of roles—ability and willingness to care for the aging, incapacitated parent
>
> Intrapsychic relationship to parental memories—effect on development

(All ages)

> Formation of cross-generational relationships—"resonance" with friends of all ages based on empathy stemming from sharing of common human experiences in the life cycle

Mentor Relationships

(Late teens and 20s)

    Choosing, relating to a mentor

    Role as a mentee—effect on work identity, creativity, role as a spouse, parent, etc.

(30s)

    Synthesizing identifications wtih the mentor, leading to emergence of personal skills and creativity

    Separating from, mourning for the mentor

    Becoming a mentor

(40s)

    Emergence as a mentor

    Reaction to creativity of mentees—facilitation vs. competitiveness and jealousy

    Ability to value and appraise creativity in others as well as the self

(50s)

    Use of power, position, prestige to facilitate mentee's development

    Ability to surrender real power to younger generation, to "pass the torch"

    Continued appropriate involvement as mentor

Relationship to Society

(Late teens and 20s)

    Polarization of real vs. idealized conceptualization of society

    Recognition of the self as part of larger structure—community, country, world

    Desire to change, improve society

    Finding a productive place in society

(30s–40s)

    Acceptance of imperfections in society and one's limited ability to change them

    Willingness to continue contributing to an imperfect world

    Balancing individual needs against those of others—the poor, etc.

(50s and beyond)

    Tolerance of change in society—adaptation to it

    Value placed on continued contribution to society

    Leadership roles in the community, philanthropic activities

Work

(Late teens and 20s)
>   Ability to make a choice, to identify work skills
>   Growth of capacity for sustained work
>   Pleasure, interest in work
>   Success and failure

(30s)
>   Solidification of work identity
>   Continued development of skills
>   Level of achievement
>   Balancing of work and family, work and play, etc.

(40s–50s)
>   Continued development of skills and achievement
>   Acceptance of failure to reach certain goals
>   Choice of new or second career—effect on development, realistic
>   or not
>   Working for society, for others
>   Use of power and position

(60s–70s)
>   Continued involvement in meaningful work and play
>   Ability to transfer power to the young
>   Attitudes toward retirement

Play

(Late teens and 20s)
>   Ability to participate and enjoy individual and group play
>   Mental and physical play—nature of, appropriateness to young-
>   adult developmental phase
>   Balancing work and play

(30s)
>   Use of play as a release—of tension, of aggression, to maintain
>   physical and emotional health
>   Play and the family—as a means of avoiding involvement or in-
>   creasing involvement—joint activities
>   Emergency of new play forms and interests

(40s, 50s, and beyond)
>   Play in relation to the developmental themes of attempted mastery
>   of time and death—e.g., chess, golf, etc.
>   Increased capacity for mental hobbies and play—reading, paint-
>   ing, music, etc.—as ability for physical play diminishes

Effect of increased leisure on play—meaningful use of time vs.
   pleasureless activity

Finances

(Late teens and 20s)
   Beginning of ability to support oneself
   Effect of prolonged financial dependence on parents
   Management of money—frivolous or careful
(30s)
   Power to earn—conflicted or not
   Use of money—to facilitate development of family and self
   Appropriateness of saving, investments
(40s–50s)
   Attitudes toward money vs. people, play, travel, etc.
   Ability to use money for present pleasure
   Planning for the future—insurance, savings, college for children,
      retirement
(60s and beyond)
   Adaptation to retirement income
   Plans for money after personal death—making a will, providing
      for spouse, children, community

CASE EXAMPLE

Identifying Information

a. Patient: R. is a 43-year-old physician. A handsome man, about
six feet tall; his graying hair, fine features, trim figure, and confident
bearing give him the air of a gracefully aging middle-aged man of emotional substance. With colleagues his gentleness, easy facility with
words, and intelligence command respect, admiration, even fear.

b. Spouse: His 40-year-old wife of 20 years, by contrast, is often
anxious and preoccupied. Slightly overweight, she pays little attention
to her appearance. A college graduate, she has been at loose ends since
their son left for college within the last year.

c. Son: Eighteen-year-old J. is a freshman at a large university. Described as bright and capable, he plans to be a physician like his father.

d. Although no one else lives in the home, the patient and his
wife are involved in the care of his elderly mother, who lives nearby.

Referral Source

The patient was self-referred. Despite his wife's encouragement and a brief positive experience with psychotherapy in his late twenties, he came for treatment with considerable reluctance.

Chief Complaint

With considerable embarrassment R. revealed, "I came to see you because of my sex life. I've started to lose interest in my wife sexually. It's depressing me and I want it to change now." By the end of the evaluation it was clear that R.'s sexual problems were not as acute as he presented them and that they had antecedents at several phases of development.

His wife asked to be seen. In a single diagnostic review she complained mildly of her husband's tendency to "work too hard and avoid me," but she talked mostly about herself. "I think maybe I'm the one who should be here, not R. I really feel lost." She was later referred for treatment of her own.

History of Present Illness

R.'s lack of interest in his wife started approximately three years ago when she "let herself go." "As she started to gain weight I started to lose interest and became impotent." At first the decreased interest led to a diminution in the frequency of intercourse from twice to once per week. The impotence occurred for the first time a year ago and now happened about a third of the time.

On occasion R. was able to overcome his sexual reluctance by fantasizing about *Playboy* centerfolds. As the frequency of intercourse diminished and the impotence increased, his wife tried to help through vigorous foreplay including previously taboo oral sex. Her efforts were moderately successful at first but increasingly of no avail.

R. summed up the current state of affairs as follows: "I'm all right as long as I don't think about her. As soon as I do I go limp so fast it makes my head spin. My God, I'm in bed with a 40-year-old woman."

Developmental History

R. was a planned child, and as far as he was able to determine, pregnancy, labor, and delivery were uneventful: A full-term infant, he weighed eight pounds. R.'s parents had wanted a girl, but as he grew and demonstrated his brightness, he became identified as the "shining light" of the family, overshadowing his older brother. A compliant, healthy infant, R. was bottle fed, and he was told he was weaned at about one year of age. Mother was involved in the care of her children on a full-time basis, and had always enjoyed her role as a mother, particularly of infants.

Toilet training commenced in the second year of life and was conducted with firmness and authority. The family enema bag was a fixture. Both parents spoke of the virtue of "being regular" and R. vividly recalled the bathroom ritual which continued until he was seven or eight, in which he would sit on the toilet and bend forward, his face in his mother's dress, as she inserted the enema nozzle in his rectum. Precocious language development—talking in sentences by 18 months—drew attention to R. Adults enjoyed him and he was nicknamed "the little genius." His mother told R. that he was an independent toddler who did not seem to mind her rare absences.

R. clearly remembered his tonsillectomy, which occurred at age five. He awoke to find his penis bandaged and bleeding—he had been circumcised at the same time without being told—and his father sitting by his bedside, "smiling like Count Dracula."

Father was often away on business during the oedipal years, and on those occasions R. slept with his mother, serving as her closest daytime companion as well. He knew he was well entrenched as "her favorite." "The sun rose and set on me."

Although he did not recall them, mother told him of frequent nightmares. His first memory of a dream was from about age eight. In it a "sinister stranger" in a flowing robe chased him around the house. Variations on this dream occurred occasionally throughout childhood and adulthood as well.

R. also remembered being invited into the bathroom by his father "to talk." As father lay in the tub with his penis floating on the water, seemingly disconnected, R. tried very hard not to look.

In the first and second grades he had a series of childhood illnesses. Consequently father discouraged physical activity out of an exaggerated concern for his health, leading to a self-imposed isolation from exercise that became a lifelong pattern.

Although outwardly R. seemed to be happy and was successful academically, elementary school was a wretched time "because of my tremendous sexual curiosity. I was sure nobody else was as curious about sex as I was." During third grade he lived in constant fear that his classmates would follow through on their threat to tell his father that they had caught him in sexual play with a neighborhood girl. R's estrangement from his peer group was a sure sign of his already prominent emotional conflicts.

In school R. was very bright and successful. His inclination for the sciences fell on deaf ears at home where his father's interests were entirely in religion and philosophy. R. attached himself to teachers and merchants who were willing to pay attention to him and teach him about radios, clocks, motors, and so on.

He ejaculated for the first time when seduced by one of these men in the storeroom of an appliance store. As an early adolescent R's mind was flooded by secret sexual thoughts about female teachers and classmates. He recalled that at age 14 he had crawled into his mother's empty bed, the covers still warm from her body heat. Later, in treatment, he revealed that he had masturbated, thinking of girls and of the back and leg rubs his mother gave him when he was a little boy. R. vehemently denied preadolescent masturbation; in fact, he was certain young children were incapable of having erections. "Little kids don't get sexually excited like that," he said. As an adolescent and young adult his frequent masturbation was accompanied by fantasies about having intercourse. Later, he revealed with great embarrassment that he sometimes had homosexual fantasies as well. By midadolescence he was isolated and lonely, separated from his peers by his intelligence and anxieties. Several moves during latency and adolescence accentuated the problem in making friends.

R. felt "absolutely liberated" when he left home for college and found himself engaged in many pleasures that he knew would displease his strict parents. Sex was only one of these. Reading new books, eating different foods, and relating to new people were others.

He began dating at 18 and had intercourse for the first time two years later. A pattern developed of impotence on the initial attempt at intercourse, followed by successful coitus.

The twenties were a period of academic achievement. R.'s acceptance to medical school filled him with confidence. "It even helped my sex life. I felt more sure of myself, I knew I had something to offer." He began to plan actively for a career in medical research. "I knew in college that I wanted to do research, but I was afraid to think about it until I got my acceptance. Once I had that I knew it could *really* happen. I looked back on my life, at all that pain during my childhood, and I just knew things were going to get better."

And they were. At 23 he married. His son was born two years later. Despite the work pressures of medical school, internship, and residency, the early years of the marriage were essentially happy ones. With practice, the young couple's sex life improved, and the anxiety about sex which was present in the first year or two of marriage disappeared. "I had turned into a pretty good stud. I even began to think I was good looking."

By 30, R. was happier than he had ever been. He was engaged in research with a prominent leader in his field who encouraged his career. His son, who seemed to be healthy and happy, was a source of great pride. After many financial lean years he was beginning to make some money, and although he worked very hard and did not have any hobbies, he and his wife had developed a small circle of friends and looked to the future with anticipation.

R. remained considerably distant from his parents. An occasional letter and rare visit were the only forms of contact he permitted despite a near-constant preoccupation with thoughts of them.

Suddenly, at 32 his life was dramatically changed when R. developed a rapidly growing malignant testicular cancer. In the midst of a nightmarish few weeks he was operated on and subjected to radiation therapy that resulted in sterilization. The course of his life was profoundly altered.

He and his wife had been attempting to have another child. R. tearfully recalled their sadness when they discovered that he was sterile. The growing sense of sexual and emotional closeness was shattered, and for three or four years distance and cautiousness characterized their relationship.

When R. was 37 his father died after a long illness. During the illness R. managed, at great emotional cost, a rapprochement with his parents. He was torn by feelings of anger and anxiety which seemed inappropriate to the reality of the situation as he watched his father slowly die. After the death he encouraged his mother to move nearby so he could take care of her.

Family History

Father: R.'s father was raised in a large farm family. His strict but loving parents were fundamentalist in their religious beliefs and actively preached these values to their children. Despite considerable academic success in high school, R.'s father had to work and could not pursue further formal learning. Moderately successful as a small businessman, he invested himself in religion and reading. Although the patient had little contact with his father after he left home, he felt that his father had lived a fairly happy but restricted life until his final illness. Father seemed pleased by the patient's success, but deeply hurt and puzzled by the sense of estrangement between them.

Mother: R.'s mother was described as a constant worrier, a "sad old lady." R. felt she was emotionally and sexually neglected by her husband and consequently centered her life on her children, particularly R., to the neglect of her own development. She staunchly took her husband's side in the quarrels with R., but after his death developed a very deep dependence on the patient. "She's smothering; sometimes I feel like she thinks I'm her child again." Mother's childhood was relatively happy. Her parents were emotionally and financially successful people, and she was attending college when she met and married R.'s father.

Older brother F: Named after his father, F. was described as "one of those plodders in life; he's done O.K., but nothing special." As a young child R. looked up to his sibling, two years older; but quickly discovered that he was brighter and more capable than his brother. They "coexisted" through much of childhood. Brother's repeated failures as an adult—in business and marriage—created a severe imbalance in their relationship. "I guess I'll end up taking care of him, as I am my mother. I think I've reached the point where I'd like to be friends with my brother, but there's nothing there. It's kind of sad."

Additional Procedures

No additional procedures were part of this diagnostic evaluation. However, a major theme in the psychotherapy was the patient's failure to pursue regular medical follow-up after his cancer surgery and radiation. This failure had a direct bearing on his current sexual functioning, since replacement doses of sexual hormones were required because of the loss of testicular hormone production resulting from the testicular surgery and irradiation.

For 11 years the patient had been immobilized by his unresolved feelings about the surgery. Only after dealing in treatment with his rage over being castrated, his inability to father another child, and the multitude of connections between this adult experience and his childhood sexual conflicts—"My father castrated me at age five [the circumcision], and it happened again 27 years later"—was he able to approach and cooperate with an endocrinologist.

Diagnosis

a. *Descriptive diagnosis:* Psychoneurosis, anxiety type, with depressive features.

b. *Dynamic formulation:* R.'s sexual symptoms were the result of an unresolved infantile neurosis exaggerated by adult experience. During the oedipal phase, maternal and paternal seductiveness in the form of frequent enemas, exaggerated interest, nudity, and sleeping together greatly stimulated R.'s infantile sexual impulses and curiosity. At the same time, the paradoxical parental preaching against sexual curiosity, and responsibility for the sexually punitive circumcision were instrumental in producing a major intrapsychic conflict over sexuality and a punitive superego. This unresolved infantile neurosis was manifested during latency by an inability to repress oedipal strivings and by an undiminished sexual curiosity. In adolescence the upsurge of sexual impulses produced by puberty led to a conscious preoccupation with incestuous wishes toward mother and homosexual fantasies and actions as a defense against them. The patient experienced intense guilt and constant anxiety throughout his adolescent years.

In young adulthood the quiescent conflict was reactivated in a major way by the testicular cancer. The resulting surgery and radiation were adult analogues of the circumcision, unconsciously representing punishment for aggressive and sexual wishes just as the circumcision was felt to be punishment for infantile sexual interests. A new dimension was added to the conflict at middle age as the patient began to react to the aging process in his wife's body (and his own), leading to a new outbreak of impotence.

Thus the infantile neurosis was the foundation of a sexual conflict that interfered with sexual development during childhood and was reactivated and added to in young adulthood by a testicular cancer and in midlife by a reaction to the aging process in his wife and himself.

c. *Developmental formulation:* R.'s infancy was characterized by consistent maternal care. Physically healthy and innately bright, he mastered most of the developmental tasks of the oral and anal phases without major difficulty and emerged from infancy as a psychologically separate, intact human being.

During the oedipal phase an intense infantile neurosis was exaggerated by parental seductiveness and punitiveness. The unresolved conflicts continued into latency, interfering with the latency tasks of repression of infantile sexuality, and the formation of comfortable peer relationships.

Adolescence was characterized by academic success, but also by the continuance of marked anxiety around sexual issues, and isolation from peers. In late adolescence the patient broke away from home but did not resolve his infantile psychological ties to his parents. He did not fully psychologically separate.

Regular heterosexual activity, which occurred belatedly, and career success elevated self-esteem in his twenties. R. engaged the young-adult developmental tasks of intimacy and parenthood with moderate success until the cancer surgery reactivated his infantile sexual conflicts, resulting in diminished sexual performance and emotional estrangement from his wife.

As he approached middle age, R. became preoccupied with the aging changes in his wife's body and his own—already imperfect because of the testicular surgery and diminished hormone production resulting from it—and discovered that his impotence and avoidance of intimacy had returned with a new intensity, precipitating a plea for treatment.

Treatment Recommendations

The patient was felt to be an excellent candidate for intensive, psychoanalytically oriented psychotherapy or psychoanalysis. Intensive, long-term treatment was indicated because the current sexual problems were deep-seated and of long standing. If they had been understood to be primarily a reflection of an adult-developmental conflict over aging, a briefer, less intense form of psychotherapy could have been recommended. Because R. was bright, verbal, and well motivated (his symptoms were seriously interfering with his sexual and emotional relationship with his wife), the prognosis was felt to be good-to-excellent.

Result

The patient was treated in psychoanalysis for four years. The analysis of his infantile sexual conflicts, the working through of his unresolved feelings of rage and mourning connected with the cancer surgery, and the resultant ability to work closely with an endocrinologist to maintain normal hormonal levels led to a disappearance of the impotence, a marked diminution in anxiety, and increased intimacy with his wife. R. was also able to begin to care for his aging mother and befriend his brother.

REFERENCES

Diagnostic and statistical manual of mental disorders III. Washington, D.C.: American Psychiatric Association, 1980.

Erikson, E. H. Eight ages of man. In *Childhood and society.* New York: W. W. Norton, 1963, pp. 247–269.

Freud, A. *Normality and pathology in childhood: Assessments of development.* New York: International Universities Press, 1965.

Kolansky, H., & Stennis, W. *A developmental history outline.* Unpublished manuscript, 1964.

Levinson, D. J., Darrow, C. N., Klein, E. B., Levinson, M. H., & McKee, B. *The seasons of a man's life.* New York: Alfred A. Knopf, 1978.

Stevenson, I. The psychiatric interview and the psychiatric examination. In S. Arieti (Ed.), *The American handbook of psychiatry.* New York: Basic Books, 1965, pp. 197–236.

Wolbert, L. *The technique of psychotherapy.* New York: Grune & Stratton, pp. 448–571.

12

The Effects of
Adult-Developmental Concepts
on Psychotherapy

In Chapter 4 we presented some basic ideas on the nature of adulthood. In this chapter we examine the implications of those ideas for psychotherapy. As an introduction to these remarks, we will consider some of the basic tenets about the developmentally oriented treatment of the adult presented in the Conference on Psychoanalytic Evaluation and Research, Commission IX report (1974).

The developmental orientation has important implications for clinical work because it provides a new framework from which to view the adult. For example, since development is considered to be a lifelong process, the patient *of any age* is understood to be in the midst of dynamic change. Since he is still developing, diagnosis and treatment focus on the current, phase-specific, adult-developmental tasks as well as the residue from earlier experiences and conflicts, thus ascribing a position of increased importance to the present and the future. Because the developmental orientation focuses on the potential for *healthy* development, it brings the *whole person* into focus as the primary interest of the therapist.

Pathology, then, is redefined as primarily deviation from normal development, an outgrowth of inadequate developmental functioning. Conflict, which is an inescapable part of all development, can produce either healthy progress or impairment and arrest.

Since development and conflict are lifelong processes, no longer confined primarily to childhood, adult development, like child development, can be arrested. *Thus the goal of treatment in the adult, as in the child, becomes not the removal of symptoms but the removal of blocks to the still evolving personality and to the course of current and future development.*

HYPOTHESIS: THE FUNDAMENTAL DEVELOPMENT ISSUES OF CHILDHOOD CONTINUE AS CENTRAL ASPECTS OF ADULT LIFE, BUT IN ALTERED FORM

Consequently the adult elaboration of such developmental themes as the oedipal complex and the separation–individuation process must be elicited as well as their childhood course. The purpose of this elaboration, which grows out of the joint therapeutic inquiry by patient and therapist, is to understand the interaction between the infantile and adult experience that resulted in interferences with past and current functioning.

The following case example, which is oversimplified to make the point, illustrates how this developmental concept may be used therapeutically.

A 35-year-old woman came for treatment after her boss, a man 25 years her senior, had broken off their affair of seven years. In a dramatic confrontation between mistress and wife, precipitated by the patient, the boss chose to remain with his spouse. The patient was shocked by his action since she genuinely and naïvely believed he preferred her.

When she was five, her father, whom she adored, left home, promising to come for her once he was settled. Throughout latency and the early adolescent years his visits diminished in frequency and eventually stopped completely. The patient lived on the secret hope that father would return one day to carry out his promise.

The oedipal implications of substituting boss for father and his spouse for mother soon became obvious to the patient, as did the connection between father's promise to take her with him and the employer's promise to marry her. However, from a developmental standpoint, this insight was only the first step in the therapeutic process. It remained for the therapist to gradually help the patient understand how her traumatic oedipal experience at age five reverberated through every succeeding phase of development, culminating in the unfulfilling adult affair. For example, in latency an intense fantasy preoccupation with father interfered with the development of friendships and hobbies. In adolescence young men were spurned because father was not there to approve of them. In her twenties she failed to engage the young-adult developmental tasks of intimacy and parenthood because of a growing attraction to older men who either ignored her or participated in brief affairs.

As enlightening as these multiphasic insights were, they too were but another step in the therapeutic process. It remained for therapist and patient to link the insights to the current developmental tasks which were arrested. For example, as the patient came to see that she had chosen her jobs on the basis of a search for a father/boss rather than a phase-appropriate interest in career advancement, she sought out a better position and upgraded her education. At age 38 she married, experiencing love and intimacy, but not parenthood. She poignantly noted that therapy was bittersweet because it showed her what she had lost as well as what she had gained.

In summary, then, the recognition that the fundamental developmental issues of childhood continue as central aspects of adult life can clarify the therapeutic task by focusing the therapist's attention on the following three goals: (1) defining the relationship between infantile experience and adult symptomatology; (2) elaborating the effects of the infantile experience on all subsequent developmental tasks, from childhood to adulthood; and (3) relating the insights to current, phase-specific arrests in development, leading to a reengagement of the adult-developmental process.

Hypothesis: The Developmental Processes in Adulthood Are Influenced by the Adult Past as well as the Childhood Past

This idea complicates the therapist's task, since significant experiences at *all* stages of the life span must be considered and evaluated *according to their affective importance and effect on subsequent development.*

The most painful memory to a 38-year-old man suffering from a neurotic depression was the loss of a job at age 25. He saw that experience as the turning point in his life, since from then on he considered himself to be a failure. The therapist's understanding of that experience as an interference with the adult-developmental task of achieving a work identity as well as an expression of a neurotic conflict with infantile determinants allowed him to emphathize with the *patient's* preoccupation with the overdetermined experience.

In the following example the patient attempted to recapture and relive his young-adult experiences. The adult past thus became a central topic in treatment.

After the death of his first wife, a 50-year-old man married a woman of 30 and began a second family. He sought treatment because of inappropriate rage at his new wife and children as expressed in his wish for his young wife's exclusive attention and his envy of her interest in their young children. The patient resented the burdens of parenthood. He had raised one family and now, in his fifties, should be free to enjoy life with his new wife.

The treatment took on intriguing dimensions as the patient explored his concurrent roles of father, grandfather, and husband. He experienced what he called "stimulus overload" as he tried to cope with his relationships with a new wife and young family and grown children and their families. In addition, these relationships would trigger powerful memories from his own childhood and young-adult years which were fascinating and draining.

By focusing on the contrast between the pleasant memories about fatherhood from early adulthood and the unpleasant ones from the present, the therapist used the adult past to help the patient come to a fuller understanding of his current developmental dilemma. Gradually, painfully, he came to see that he had married a much younger woman and begun a second family in an attempt to compensate for his fears of aging and diminished potency. His magical attempt to reverse the aging process by becoming a father had left him again with the very real burdens and responsibilities of parenthood at a time when he wished to be free of them. He came to recognize, however, that he had charted a course for the remainder of his life which ensured an active life, filled with people who lived and needed him.

HYPOTHESIS: DEVELOPMENT IN ADULTHOOD, AS IN CHILDHOOD, IS DEEPLY INFLUENCED BY THE BODY AND PHYSICAL CHANGE

Because adult development is deeply influenced by the body and physical change, it is incumbent on the therapist to continually assess the patient's thoughts and feelings about bodily appearance, functioning, and aging. These attitudes are repeatedly avoided because of the narcissistic injury involved and may not be brought into the treatment unless the therapist is aware of the powerful resistances against them. The therapist may need to actively lead the exploration of feelings about the body, bodily care, exercise, and so on, particularly in those instances in which there is a question of possible organic disease. Appropriate therapeutic intervention may include referral and consultation with medical specialists and active evaluation and exploration of the results with the patient.

A woman of 38 avoided seeing a cardiologist despite the presence of symptoms (occasional missed beats and an arrhythmia) because of her strong belief that the symptoms were psychological. She did indeed have a cardiac neurosis, based in part on the death of her mother from a heart attack and a serious operation of her own, both at about age 10. She subsequently developed an anxious preoccupation with bodily functioning and a profound fear of physicians. After the establishment of a therapeutic alliance and an extended period of work on the cardiac neurosis, the patient was able, at the therapist's suggestion, to see a cardiologist. The confirmation of definite but controllable organic disease led to a marked increase in cardiac anxiety and major reworking of the infantile factors in the cardiac neurosis, including her rage at her parents (and in the transference, the therapist) for subjecting her to the operation (and to the adult cardiac evaluation).

That work was followed by an exploration of the ways in which the patient had avoided caring for her body (exercise, checkups, etc.) and experiencing its pleasures (sexual inhibitions).

Neglect of the adult body in treatment may grow out of the *therapist's* need to avoid the issue. Since therapy is done mainly by people in their thirties, forties, and beyond, therapist and patient are often trying to master the same feelings about bodily decline.

HYPOTHESIS: A CENTRAL, PHASE-SPECIFIC THEME OF ADULT DEVELOPMENT IS THE NORMATIVE CRISIS PRECIPITATED BY THE RECOGNITION AND ACCEPTANCE OF THE FINITENESS OF TIME AND THE INEVITABILITY OF PERSONAL DEATH

If the therapist appreciates the centrality and power of the twin themes of the finiteness of time and the inevitability of personal death in the physic life of his adult patients, therapeutic techniques to deal with them must follow. We are not speaking only of morbid or even pathological focusing on time and death, but of the *universal* power of adult preoccupations with these themes.

In the past these midlife feelings have been seen primarily as "precipitants," "situational factors," or "derivatives of earlier conflicts"— which they are. But in addition they are major forces in their own right which act as developmental stimulants and sources of conflict as well.

Because of the narcissistic pain associated with them (just as with the adult body), thoughts and feelings about time and death are either avoided by patients or mentioned peripherally. If there is a lack of conceptual clarity as to their importance on the part of the therapist or a reluctance, comparable to the patient's, to consider such thoughts and feelings, they may never become part of the therapeutic process. In almost all instances in our experience, adult patients will sooner or later make reference to thoughts of time and limitation and personal death. It is then that the therapist, equipped with the adult-developmental theoretical armamentarium, will sensitively begin to explore them.

An analogy may be drawn between the adolescent's avoidance of sexual material and the middle-aged or older individual's avoidance of thoughts and feelings about time and death. Both are highly sensitive, well defended, and of central importance.

> A highly successful man of 43 came to treatment because of an exaggerated response to minor surgery. He was convinced that he was seriously ill and significantly limited his activities long after any restriction was appropriate. Important infantile factors were undue parental anxiety about any illness, particularly a tonsillectomy at age five, and exaggerated investment in his athletic achievements, thus establishing the body as a major focus for narcissistic gratification and vulnerability.
>
> The area became accessible after the therapist responded to the patient's joking reference to his adolescent sons. "Those bastards, they have it all in front of them. You and I are over the hill." When the therapist took the remark seriously and empathized with the powerful envy it conveyed, a torrent of words and feelings poured forth.
>
> At the time the patient was considering abandoning a highly successful career ("I want to do something great, something I'll be remembered for after I die.") and his marriage ("My wife's body is old and flabby; it disgusts me.") in a frenzied attempt to deal with his fears of aging. The therapy gradually centered on the analysis of those issues, with the eventual disappearance of the symptoms and integration of a more realistic body image.

Again, the goal of treatment is not the elimination of symptoms, but the removal of blocks to development and the integration of phase-specific developmental themes.

DEVELOPMENTAL RESONANCE

If they are linked to what we call "developmental resonance," many of the specific adult-developmental themes just discussed become particularly relevant for the therapist of any age. Empathy is understood to be an essential ingredient in the therapeutic process. Therapists are ineffective without the capacity to feel what their patients feel, to envision themselves in the patient's place. The developmental framework adds a new dimension to the meaning of empathy by demonstrating how patient and therapist are alike in that they share the same developmental continuum. Both must deal with the same developmental themes in childhood (infantile sexuality, separation from parents, learning, etc.) and adulthood (adult sexuality, work, aging, etc.). Yet they are different because each has had unique individual experiences, and *in most instances they will not be at the same point* on the developmental continuum.

Developmental resonance is the therapeutic capacity to share, respect, understand, and value the thoughts and feelings of patients of *all* ages because of explicit awareness on the part of the therapist that he either has experienced or likely will experience what his patient is feeling and living. He can appreciate and convey the same genuine interest and understanding to the five-year-old who complains of being small and powerless and to the 19-year-old who doubts his masculinity because his chest is hairless and his penis small. Although he may be younger than the 40-year-old who is pained by his baldness and wrinkles, or the 70-year-old who is painfully aware of the failure of his body to respond to his commands as it used to, he knows he is not immune to their experience or pain. The universal theme that affects all—including the therapist—is the vulnerability underlying the constantly changing body as it develops in the first half of life and regresses in the second. This example can be multiplied many times over in regard to other aspects of development.

Reference

Conference on Psychoanalytical Education and Research. Commission IX, "Child Analysis." New York: American Psychoanalytic Association, 1974.

13

Psychotherapeutic Technique and Development

In this chapter we address the effect of adult-developmental concepts on psychotherapeutic technique. A developmental orientation can change the therapist's understanding of the purpose, process, and results of his work with patients, leading to a broader and more complex conceptualization of psychotherapy.

To set the stage for the discussion, let us reiterate some of the basic clinical ideas presented in the last chapter, this time in the form of a quote from the Conference on Psychoanalytic Education and Research, Commission IX report (1974).

> The implications of the developmental orientation for clinical work stem from the view of individual human development as a continuous and life-long process. One important part of this longitudinal view is the conceptualization of mental illness not in the medical model of disease entities affecting a fully developed organ system, but in the model of functional disturbances which not only impair the current functioning of the individual but impede the development of still-evolving psychic structure and function in one or more of its lines or aspects. By placing mental illness within the broader context of the ongoing process of development, we emphasize that the aim of treatment is to enable development to proceed in all of its dimensions. This viewpoint keeps in the foreground the awareness that one is treating a person, not an illness. (p. 14)

There are other advantages to viewing the individual as still developing.

> The longitudinal view of the patient as still developing has a further advantage. It focuses on the formation of psychic structure *in process* and underscores the contiguity of normal and pathologic outcomes. Psychopathology is thus understood in terms of psychogenetic and psychodynamic devia-

225

tions from normal development and the route of reversibility in treatment is highlighted. *We treat not syndromes but developmentally arrested human beings, who have through their own defensive activity participated in the formation of their pathology and must in the same way participate in its undoing.* (pp. 14-15, italics added)

Since the publication of the Commission IX report, the person most responsible for describing the effect of the developmental orientation on clinical work with adults has been Morton Shane, an adult and child psychoanalyst. In a series of germinal papers (1977, 1979, in press), he addressed himself to many aspects of technique. In this chapter we present a number of his basic ideas, adding and elaborating with thoughts and clinical examples of our own. In our opinion, these ideas—which grew out of clinical psychoanalysis and dynamically oriented psychotherapy—have a broad application to all forms of therapeutic intervention from crisis intervention and brief psychotherapy to long-term therapy and analysis.

THE THERAPEUTIC SETTING AND THE BASIC METHOD OF FREE ASSOCIATION

The adult must learn how to free-associate. It is often assumed that the adult patient, simply because he is an adult, can instantly and automatically free-associate. Such is not the case. As with all abilities, free association must be learned, a *process* that takes many weeks or months. Usually this capacity grows as treatment progresses, so that the patient *leaves* treatment with a new and powerful introspective tool.

There are practical implications to this development conceptualization of free association, beginning with how Freud's "basic rule" is communicated to the patient. First, the term "basic rule" has limitations because it may be taken as a command and become the focus of early apprehension or resistance. It is better to speak to the patient about the "necessity of learning the method of free association." Addressing the patient's ego, we invite him to participate with us in a unique and novel adventure into his mental life and behavior *with the purpose of gaining an in-depth understanding of how his mind has developed to this point in his life.*

In keeping with this developmental approach, the therapist may frequently need, particularly during the opening and middle phases of treatment, to help the patient understand the resistances and blocks to free association which are an inevitable and continual part of the process. For example, a sophisticated mental-health worker came to treatment with a clear understanding that free association meant the verbalization of *all* thoughts without consideration as to their importance. Soon, however, without any recognition of the contradiction involved, the patient began to disregard certain associations as "unimportant." After this contradiction was pointed out, patient and analyst began to pay attention to these "unimportant" associations, leading eventually to the discovery that the patient was avoiding feelings of being an "unimportant" third child. In addition to the specific insight gained, the patient came to recognize how difficult free association was and to work with the analyst in analyzing the resistances to the process. As this work proceeded the patient began to monitor and comment on his increasing ability to associate.

When both therapist and patient understand the process involved in learning how to free-associate, neither becomes frustrated. The therapist conceptualizes his role as one of helping the patient increase the *capacity* to free-associate and does not become annoyed when a patient cannot associate as well as the therapist would like. Similarly, the patient is less likely to feel inadequate when unable to associate. The difficulty becomes an opportunity.

The developmental orientation also suggests that the modes of communication between adult patient and therapist may be broadened. To quote Shane (1977):

> I would like to suggest that an approach which encourages and accepts all modes of communication has value for the treatment of a patient of any age. A rationale is thus provided for looking at a picture drawn by an adult patient, for examining his work of art if presented in an hour, for not inadvertently discouraging his gestures, for accepting the drawing of a dream image, or even for viewing the spontaneous playful enactment as within the realm of this expanded developmental view of free association. (p. 97)

For example, Shane describes how he asked a female patient in her middle forties to "put into words *rather than* action her silent stroking of my wall" (p. 97). Various other nonverbal activities such as stroking her hair, rubbing her upper lip, and rubbing the couch also occurred. These actions had meaning for the therapist:

> Using a developmental orientation, one that conceptualizes her lack of verbalization not merely as defense but also as an arrest along developmental lines of cognitive attainment and self-object differentiation, *I learned not*

to adhere to a theory that would discourage action in order to augment verbalization; instead I encouraged her to report what she was feeling and thinking at the same time that she was involved in the action. (p. 97, italics added)

As a further example, Shane explains his response to a late-adolescent analytic patient who asked if he could bring to his hour an acclaimed film he had made in cinema class. The analyst agreed.

> He then brought a projector to his hour, showed me the film, and then lay on the couch and further associated to having shown it to me, to his thoughts about my response and so forth. I felt nothing was lost by this procedure and in fact I gained an additional input as to the affective life of my patient reflected in a non-verbal but symbolic mode. My own empathic response to his artistic production added a dimension to my private understanding of his object longing, which subsequently I was able to communicate to him. (p. 98)

So it is clear that nonverbal communications can be quite important in the treatment process and the source of meaningful insights when they are understood developmentally. However, if the patient is confronted with his nonverbal communications without understanding their value as a tool for insight he may feel confused and criticized.

An example of a well-timed therapeutic utilization of a nonverbal gesture follows.

> In anxious moments a patient would persistently run his hand through his hair, shedding dandruff on the furniture in the process. Occasionally he made passing reference to his behavior but without understanding of its meaning. Recognizing that the gesture had meaning, the therapist explained to the patient that the gesture was a form of communication that needed to be understood. The unconscious meaning of the behavior became clearer in a session marked by increasing shedding and repeated references to his father's insecurities about money and position. When the patient began associating to his father's baldness the therapist chose to connect the associations and the behavior. The patient then remembered his childhood fear of his father's bald head, which now symbolically represented father's insecurities and anxiety-ridden state. The patient's behavior was a communication that meant, "You see, I'm not like my father. I have hair." This man's lifelong struggle against identification (Greenson, 1967) now became clear with the realization that much of his behavior was based on a fear of ending up like father. Unconsciously he demonstrated his wish to be different each time he stroked his hair.

> Another patient, in his thirties, frequently made puzzling, sweeping concave gestures with his hands to illustrate his points. The therapist wondered about the meaning of these gestures, but initially could not relate them to the patient's situation. In a session following the birth of his second child, the patient talked somewhat intellectually about the birth

of his own sibling. Concurrently the concave sweep of the hands increased in frequency and seemed to closely approximate the arc of a pregnant belly. When the therapist mentioned his hunch, the patient recalled his mother's pregnant belly and expressed his wonderment at the birth process and his rage at his sibling's birth. This exploration of his identification with his pregnant mother, expressed initially through his gesture which was accepted and recognized by the therapist, greatly facilitated the treatment.

Shane (1977) reminds us that:

> While we accept the fact that children are *developmentally* incapable of communicating symbolically in words alone, we often fail to realize that many adults, who are nonetheless analyzable, may share this incapacity to varying degrees and at different times. (p. 98)

THE THERAPEUTIC WORKING ALLIANCE

Entering the Working Alliance

The term *working alliance* refers to the relatively nonneurotic, rational rapport that the patient develops with his therapist (Greenson, 1967). Because of the patient's motivation for change, sense of helplessness, conscious and rational willingness to cooperate, and ability to follow the lead of the therapist, an alliance is formed between the patient's reasonable ego and the therapist's analyzing ego (Sterba, 1934). As the patient identifies with the therapist's approach he gradually increases his capacity to participate effectively in the alliance on his own behalf.

It is often said that if a patient cannot enter into a working alliance, treatment is not possible. However, as with free association, it cannot be reasonably expected that adult or child comes to treatment prepared to immediately enter into a smooth, well-working therapeutic alliance.

The ability to utilize the therapeutic alliance is related to the attainment of maturity along the development line (A. Freud, 1965) of caring for the self. If the therapist has the unwarranted expectation that his adult patients come fully motivated for treatment, he may be unable to make the necessary therapeutic interventions to ensure emergence of the alliance. Attention to the state of the working alliance is important in all forms of therapeutic intervention. In crisis intervention the formation of an immediate therapeutic alliance is essential. In brief psychotherapy the therapist must utilize the patient's pain, sense of helplessness, and rational desire to change in order to maximize the effect of his interventions.

Generally, in exploratory therapy, the working alliance must be explained, observed, and analyzed as it develops. With relatively well-functioning neurotic patients, most aspects of the alliance are understood and integrated during the opening phase of treatment. Such is not the case with borderline or narcissistic patients, whose severe problems with trust, ego boundaries, and sense of self continually distort the reality aspects of the relationship to the therapist. In fact, building and maintaining a functional working alliance is a major therapeutic goal with narcissistic and borderline patients. Thus for *most* patients the capacity to understand and utilize the working relationship is something that develops throughout the course of treatment and undergoes continual refinement by both therapist and patient.

> A middle-aged, borderline man came for treatment after a disheartening experience with a previous therapist who had been verbally abusive and abruptly dismissed the patient as unsuitable for treatment. Because of that experience and his underlying problems with trust, he constantly distorted the *realities* of the therapeutic relationship. The patient constantly tested the therapist's feelings about him and attempted to win favor through gifts, verbal praise, and overpaying bills. Before any interpretation or clarification was made, even in the later stages of the treatment, the therapist *first* had to assess the strength of the therapeutic alliance at that moment. It was not possible to overcome the severe arrests along the developmental lines of trust and caring for the self, but the recognition of these arrests allowed the therapist to be exquisitely sensitive to the fragility of the working alliance and treat the patient.

Outside Motivation

Just as the developmentally oriented therapist is not distressed by his patient's limited ability to communicate verbally, neither is he unnecessarily discouraged when he discovers that the patient's motivation for treatment is strongly influenced by others. This is usually the case with children, but is often true of adults as well. For instance, in the individual therapy of adults with marital difficulties, the working alliance may be strengthened *or* threatened by third parties. The spouse can become a psychological ally or a bitter enemy who feels left out in the cold. If the therapist understands marriage as a developmental process leading to an increased capacity for intimacy, it is easy for him to empathize with the spouse who views therapy as a threat. Utilizing these developmental concepts, Shane (1977) describes the following clinical situation:

> ... a 22 year old woman, who had been in analysis for two years prior to her marriage, found herself with a phase-appropriately, as well as neurotically, jealous husband on her hands when she wished to continue the analysis after marriage. Her husband threatened to withhold all financial support. *Using a developmental approach I was able to help her focus on understanding both her husband's jealously [sic] and her own neurotic and phase-appropriate disloyalty conflicts between husband and analyst. This required more than uncovering the genetic roots of her distress; it was also necessary to confront her with her conflicted but phase-appropriate wish for an exclusive intimacy with her husband.*
> I agreed to see her husband for one visit. Although the interview never took place, my agreement alleviated some of his suspiciousness and his fear that I jealously guarded an exclusive relationship with his wife. (p. 100, italics added)

In a clinical situation of our own, similar dynamics played a part, only this time in reverse; the patient was male and his wife experienced feelings of jealousy, rage, and depression in response to her husband's refusal to discuss his treatment.

> This 25-year-old man had been in treatment for several months when the following occurred. His wife was becoming increasingly depressed, as evidenced by crying spells and sleepless nights. When the therapist asked about her complaints the patient replied with characteristic intellectual blandness, "She feels left out in the cold; she doesn't know what goes on here." The therapist inquired further and discovered that the patient had barely mentioned therapy to his wife. He had kept her in the dark, assuming that he was not to talk about therapy with *anyone*. "I'm strictly adhering to the rules," he said. The therapist, understanding this withholding as part of the patient's problems with intimacy, focused on the rigid and isolating behavior.
> The patient responded by discussing his father's similar treatment of his mother. Gradually the patient began to share information with his wife, leading to a lifting of her depression and a heightened degree of closeness between them. The treatment, which was in danger of being sabotaged by an angry spouse, continued on a firmer footing.

Outside Information

In most descriptions of exploratory psychotherapies the utilization of information from a source other than the patient is advised against as a possible contaminant of the treatment process. That need not be the case, for the noncritical presentation of outside information can aid the process of self-observation and further the working alliance. Shane feels that the therapist should be able to utilize outside information with adults as well as children without damaging the working alliance. An example of our own illustrates the point.

> A patient in his thirties frequently procrastinated over his insurance forms, leading to delays in reimbursement. At one point the therapist was contacted by the insurance company and informed about the patient's erratic handling of the forms. The therapist in a noncritical, objective fashion described the information he had received, suggesting that here was some new information that could be understood by patient and therapist working together. A transference paradigm was revealed which indicated that the patient was unconsciously trying to get the therapist and the insurance company to care for him and clean up his messes after him, as his mother once did. The patient's increased understanding of this type of behavior had great ramifications for him since he experienced considerable resentment from his wife and colleagues for similar behavior.

TRANSFERENCE AND THE DEVELOPMENTAL APPROACH

Greenson (1967) feels that the development of psychoanalytic technique (and by extension, dynamic psychotherapy) has primarily emerged from knowledge of transference, which he defines as follows:

> By transference we refer to a special kind of relationship toward a person; it is a distinctive type of object relationship. The main characteristic is the experience of feelings to a person which do not befit that person and which actually apply to another. Essentially a person in the present is reacted to as though he were a person in the past. Transference is a repetition, a new edition of an old object relationship . . . . It is an anachronism, an error in time. A displacement has taken place; impulses, feelings, and defenses pertaining to a person in the past have been shifted onto a person in the present. It is primarily an unconscious phenomenon and the person reacting with transference feelings is in the main unaware of the distortion. (pp. 151-152)

By applying developmental principles to transference, we increase both the complexity of the phenomena and the potential for deeper understanding. Consider again the idea of transference as a new edition of the past. From a developmental standpoint, that new edition does not emanate solely from the childhood past but results from a complex, multidimensional past (i.e., the life cycle—infancy, childhood, adolescence, young adulthood). Furthermore, the new edition is constructed by the mind of the present. What is presented to us is the past as interpreted by the patient's mind in the present.

In many instances the situation is further complicated by the fact that the parents of childhood are still alive and influential in their grown children's lives. They have become the parents of adulthood. These current, real relationships affect transference. Shane writes (1977):

> Transference, and particularly the transference neurosis, while involving crucial and pathogenic elements from the past displaced on to the present, does not involve the past *exclusively*. In fact, the potency of primary objects to elicit powerful developmental conflicts in the present (albeit with strong reverberations to the repressed past) is seen throughout adolescence and indeed into adult life. (p. 102)

Among Shane's examples of such interaction are the following two:

> A young adult woman patient expressed guilt at being prettier than my wife, who represented for her a displacement from her mother not only in the past, but in the present. Her mother, an infantile and still quite attractive woman, would become distraught in true "Snow White" fashion at anyone's suggestion that her daughter was prettier than she. The patient's guilty conflict in response is in the present, the superego and oedipal roots of this conflict deep in the past notwithstanding.

> A 40 year old man visited his father after not having seen him for 25 years. Upon relating to his father his current business successes, my patient was dismayed by the bitter, jealous response: "Some people have all the luck." His son reacted with a disastrous episode of gambling on the stock market. *Both my patient and I were impressed by the power his father still possessed to evoke in him unconscious superego punishment.* Similar wishes to please, to ingratiate and to submit were displaced from his father on to me, partly from his past and partly from a current phase-appropriate attempt to mourn the loss of a still longed-for protecting father. (p. 102, italics added)

New Transference Uses of the Therapist

Adult-developmental theory brings with it the recognition that the adult patient may use the therapist as a transference object in ways that were not possible in childhood.

A prime example would be a son or daughter transference. Although children in treatment play at being parents and assign the role of child to the therapist, it is not possible to transfer feelings about real children without first becoming a parent—an adult experience. In some instances, particularly with an older patient and a younger therapist, a son or daughter transference may be central to the therapeutic alliance and to an understanding of the patient.

A woman in her early fifties came for brief psychotherapy because of her pain as she watched her 23-year-old son struggle to leave home. The therapist's explanation of his *continued* search for identity—a task she felt he should have finished in his teens—relieved her fears that he was severely disturbed, and stimulated her transference relationship to the therapist. Her son's verbal abuse and rudeness, a defense against dependency, contrasted sharply with the therapist's kindness, understanding, and empathy, and led to the emergence of a transference paradigm in which the therapist was seen as a good and caring son. This idealization facilitated the exploration of the *mother's* role in her son's conflict—namely, ambivalence about giving him up.

At that point the therapist became the equivalent of an adult transitional object facilitating the mother's separation from the son. As the son actually individuated, the patient regressively tried to reestablish the relationship in the transference through attempts to control the therapist and seduce him around issues of medication and a mutual interest in literature ("Let's read Chaucer, why talk about such depressing stuff.").

The resolution of the transference allowed the patient to focus on other phase-specific developmental issues such as the "empty-nest syndrome"—what to do with life now that her children were raised—as well as her changing relationship with her husband, and so on. In the process the therapist went from being "my good son" to "my good friend."

This material also illustrates the concept of developmental resonance since the therapist was able to empathize with the experiences of the son and the mother and *make both sets of feelings understandable to her.* His appreciation of the dynamic conflict of both—at different points on the life cycle but locked in an intense, mutual struggle against separation—was the basis for the therapeutic interaction between therapist and patient. This example also illustrates the point that transference, "essentially a person in the present is reacted to as though he were a person in the past" (Greenson, 1967, p. 1511), is not limited to analysis or intensive psychotherapy. Not only is it a part of all therapeutic relationships, but of all human relationships as well. What differs in treatment is the therapist's understanding and recognition of transference, and his ability to utilize it to further his therapeutic goals, whether they be primarily support, insight, or interpretation.

RESISTANCE, DEFENSE, AND DEVELOPMENT

The concept of phase-specific and phase-appropriate defenses has proved enormously useful for the dynamic clinician (A. Freud, 1965).

Vaillant (1971) has conceptualized a particularly useful scheme of placing the mechanisms of defense along developmental lines:

1. Primitive defenses: denial, projection, reality distortion
2. Neurotic defenses: repression, isolation, undoing, etc.
3. Mature defenses: sublimation, suppression, humor, etc.

By utilizing a developmental perspective in regard to defenses, as described by Vaillant, the therapist has a powerful tool in that he can better organize and select his response to the patient's defenses. It is generally agreed that resistances and defenses are selectively interpreted in exploratory therapy and strengthened or left untouched in supportive forms of therapy. How does the therapist decide when to intervene? Our contention is that the clear identification of phase-specific and phase-appropriate defenses helps in the selection procedure. Basically, phase-appropriate defenses are interpreted less often than more primitive and maladaptive defenses. As Shane (1977) states:

> Since developmental phases continue into adult life, phase appropriate, developmentally appropriate, defenses should be, by the same token, respected in the adult. For example, a pregnant woman's narcissistic regression might not be interpreted unless it were pathologically excessive. Empathetic identifications and selective regressions in the developmental process of parenthood would be similarly assessed for their phase-appropriateness. The analyst of the adult needs to consider the injunction so prevalent in the analysis of children to not interfere unduly with normally progressing development. (pp. 103-104)

In a similar way, utilizing developmental principles, the therapist is better able to distinguish between resistance and unavoidable developmental tasks. If the therapist does not distinguish between resistance and interferences that are developmentally based, he opens himself to charges of rigidity and insensitivity.

Nowhere is this fact clearer than in therapeutic work with graduate and postgraduate students. Take, for example, the medical student. Medical training requires the absorption of incredible amounts of information, often in stressful situations involving life and death. The therapist must appreciate this stress and be willing at a moment's notice to actively change and adapt his reality, that is, frequency and time of appointments, to the need of his student-patient. Anything less than a complete understanding and flexible response to the developmental stresses upon the student will be experienced by the student-patient as a gross lack of empathy and may lead to the premature disruption of therapy. In the past we may have regarded some of these stress variables as simply "situational." In counterdistinction, the developmental approach places these stresses and demands in the forefront of the therapist's attention and encourages a broad, complex approach in which they are not automatically viewed as resistances to treatment but are appreciated as part of the patient's evolving personality and essential current and future life tasks.

RECONSTRUCTIONS

Reconstructions, the deductions of patient and therapist about important events and feelings that must have occurred in the patient's past, have always played an important role in exploratory therapy. In recent years, Kohut (1971) has ascribed increased importance to empathic reconstructions in therapy. Thinking developmentally is a great help to the clinician in reconstructing the patient's unique life experiences. After some experience with a patient it is often possible to deduce from a sense of *omission*, from what has been left out, what has been repressed.

The nature of the reconstruction that the therapist presents depends upon the depth of understanding of normal development that he has. This basic knowledge is important for every therapist so that his reconstructions will convey a ring of truth to the patient. This sense of conviction is realized by the patient when the reconstruction fits like an important piece of a jigsaw puzzle, adding clarity and completion to the patient's life history. Once the reconstruction has occurred, its effect reverberates throughout the patient's life cycle as the new insight is applied to all phases of the patient's life. The patient thus experiences a sense of *continuity* about his life in the past and the present.

A patient, who himself was a therapist, found himself becoming anxious and annoyed when his own patients talked about their siblings. He could not understand his response. Another problem area for him was separations. He had been very homesick when he went to camp as a teen-ager and even when he went away to college. As an adult he had refused to consider postgraduate training in some excellent centers because they were "across the country, in another universe."

Gradually it became clear that the patient had walled off strong feelings about his older brother's accidental death when the patient was seven years old, since he spoke of the tragedy only occasionally, and then in a casual, offhand manner. Using his knowledge of child development and the patient's history, the therapist reconstructed that the patient, as a young child of seven, must have been frightened by the funeral and terrified by his mother's emotional collapse, which included a hospitalization. His own conflicted feelings about his brother, which likely included pleasure at the brother's death, were so powerful that they were repressed—hence the sense of casualness—but they continued to dominate his unconscious life and were expressed consciously ever since in his fear of leaving home. Probably as a seven-year-old he expected that the same thing would happen to him if he left home, as punishment for his death wishes. The ring of conviction came from *his* adding to the reconstruction the up-to-then incidental fact that his brother's death had occurred when he went away from home for the first time on his own, soon after he learned to drive.

A flood of feelings was released by the reconstruction, which led to a reworking of many aspects of his attitudes about his own aggression, and to a diminution of the symptoms.

COUNTERTRANSFERENCE

The developmental orientation implies that not only the patient but the therapist as well is in a state of continuous, dynamic flux and change. Although in one of his last papers, *Analysis Terminable and Interminable,* Freud (1937) suggested that analysts consider reanalysis every five years, implying a process of continuous crisis and growth, there is often considerable individual resistance to this concept. Some patients, and also therapists, expect the therapist to be a shining example of a stable, nonchanging, completely developed individual since he presents himself as a "helpmate" to others. The reality of change and crisis in the therapist's life such as divorce, death of loved ones, or physical illness is often an important factor in the psychotherapeutic situation and the mental life of the therapist.

Generally, *countertransference* is thought of as a neurotic therapeutic response in which the patient is unconsciously misidentified with a significant and conflict-laden object from the therapist's past. Once such countertransference feelings are recognized, the therapist should alter his response through self-analysis or treatment. In addition, the therapist's feelings and reactions may provide the basis for a more empathic understanding of the patient's feelings, as well as a heightened appreciation of the unconscious meanings of his conflicts.

An addition to the above description of countertransference is contained in a paper by Shane (in press) in which he describes the unanticipated personal and developmental gain that may accrue to the therapist from his work with a patient:

> By the same token, neurotic conflicts discerned by the analyst in his countertransference responses to a specific patient may carry with them developmental arrests and lags which also require *working through* if only in self analysis. Such efforts on the part of the analyst should further the (inevitably) incomplete work of his training—(and subsequent self) analysis. There is thus unanticipated developmental gain that may accrue to the analyst indirectly through work with a patient. By a defensive-adaptive mechanism of active to passive (applying to the self what is applied to the patient), or through empathy, amelioration of the analyst's own difficulties via mutual influences between patient and analyst can transpire alongside of the patient's improvement. (p. 196)

Shane also describes a process that occurs in therapists during their careers which is related to the evolution and working through of their mentor relationships. A necessary developmental step for each therapist is to slowly free himself from the onetime necessary idealizations and identifications with mentors' standards and practices. Countertransference reactions, in this broader sense, may arise when a therapist, because of unconscious identification with former mentors, slavishly applies the same practices. In describing a countertransference reaction of his own, Shane wrote of his need to use the couch, to do "real" analysis, as he thought his own analyst would have done, with a patient who would have benefited from psychoanalysis using a face-to-face parameter.

> I struggle against my desire to do "real analysis"; my clinical judgement says that all will go better if she continues in the sitting up position. I struggle, too, with the developmental limitation within myself of doing work which does not meet the standards of my own less than realistic, partly unconscious, ego ideal, forged in transference idealization of my own analyst, of Freud, and of the profession of psychoanalysis itself. These attitudes I have struggled with and have attempted to correct in my own thinking and writing, but I can see them still, reflected in my work with this patient. The developmental lag within "analysthood" may not be countertransference in the narrow sense; however, I think it falls roughly within *that* sector of the analytic relationship. In this vignette I present not a problem solved but a problem I continue to struggle with. (p. 208)

In summation, the developmental approach brings into focus countertransference reactions which are complex and multilayered and thus difficult to eradicate by single acts of self-analysis. These more global countertransference feelings and reactions need to be worked through by the therapist, and therein lies the potential for considerable growth and development, particularly of professional identity. The myth of the completely trained graduate therapist who is a finished product should give way, within the developmental perspective, to a view of the therapist as a creative individual undergoing continuous growth and change in his role. Each patient offers the therapist an opportunity to work through core conflicts and aspects of professional identity.

Termination

Among the criteria that are commonly used to determine readiness for termination are symptom relief, structural change, transference resolution, and improvement in self-esteem. The developmental approach adds one important dimension and criterion, namely, the elimination of blocks to development. Has the patient demonstrated the capacity to resume normal development and engage phase-appropriate life tasks? *It is our contention that the idea of the resumption of normal development is a broader notion that underlies the other criteria of symptom relief, structural change, transference resolution, and improvement in self-esteem.* The following case illustrated this concept.

> A young woman in her middle twenties came to treatment because of vague feelings of marital dissatisfaction, including sexual dysfunction. Over the course of her treatment she was able to resolve her feelings of narcissistic competition with men and come to accept her dependency needs. The resolution of these issues, among others, helped her lower the barriers to intimacy with her husband. Her feelings of self- and marital satisfaction improved dramatically, and in a planned fashion she terminated treatment. A number of months after treatment terminated she became pregnant and with much enjoyment had her first child. From communications to her therapist it was clear that she had made considerable strides in resolving problems with intimacy and that *the therapy had left her in a position to move on to the new developmental step of pregnancy and motherhood.*

The developmental approach places a new light on the importance of issues of separation, loss, mourning, and new adaptation in relation to termination. These issues are particularly highlighted because of an understanding of the separation-individuation process which begins in early childhood with the mother-child relationship and continues throughout the life cycle. At each phase development implies some loss, including regression, as well as progression and achievement. However, the developmental psychotherapist feels that the emotional understanding and experience of the processes involved in loss, mourning, and new internalizations are essential to both growth and increased capacity for self-observation and -differentiation. Technically, then, he will search out every opportunity to explore the patient's unique experiences with loss. Rather than avoid issues of separation, such as his own vacation or interruptions due to physical illness, he will actively place such experiences in the forefront of therapy so as to "mine the transference gold" contained in them.

Finally, the developmental approach truly captures the spirit of Freud's suggestion in *Analysis Terminable and Interminable* of the consideration of ongoing treatment at different stages of life. The door to the consulting room is never finally closed; rather, termination is more flexible and open-end. Since the resumption of normal development is the overriding goal of therapy, this flexibility implies that normative crises and transitions are to be expected after the individual leaves treatment and engages new developmental tasks. For each individual patient, the therapist must find a way in the termination process to convey to his patient that yes, certain developmental goals have been achieved during the hard work of therapy, but certainly more experiences are ahead of the patient and the therapist stands ready to participate in furthering the patient's development should the patient wish to consult him, however briefly.

REFERENCES

Conference on Psychoanalytic Education and Research. Commission IX, "Child Analysis." New York: American Psychoanalytic Association, 1974.

Freud, A. *Normality and pathology in childhood: Assessments of development.* New York: International Universities Press, 1965.

Freud, S. *Analysis terminable and interminable.* Standard edition, 23:209. London: Hogarth Press, 1937.

Greenson, R. *The technique and practice of psychoanalysis.* New York: International Universities Press, 1967.

Kohut, H. *The analysis of the self.* New York: International Universities Press, 1971.

Shane, M. A rationale for teaching analytic technique based on a developmental orientation and approach. *International Journal of Psycho-Analysis*, 1977, *58*, 95.

Shane, M. The developmental approach to "working through" in the analytic process. *International Journal of Psycho-Analysis*, 1979, *60*, 375.

Shane, M. Countertransference and the developmental approach. In *Psychoanalysis and contemporary thought.* In press.

Sterba, R. F. The fate of the ego in analytic therapy. *International Journal of Psycho-Analysis*, 1934, *15*, 117.

Vaillant, G. E. Theoretical hierarchy of adaptive ego mechanisms: A 30 year follow-up of 30 men selected for psychological health. *Archives of General Psychiatry*, 1971, *24*, 107.

14

Clinical Applications

AN ADULT-DEVELOPMENTAL APPROACH TO HYSTERICAL PSYCHOPATHOLOGY[1]

Gail Sheehy begins *Passages* (1974) by describing the origin of anxiety and depression at age 35. She reconstructs the precipitating trauma—a close call with death in Ireland—and its metamorphosis into a full-blown phobic neurosis, an irrational fear of flying. Soon thereafter her neurotic compromise failed and she experienced emotional lability, depression, and anxiety, for which barbiturates and mood elevators were prescribed. The culmination was an hallucinatory episode with conversion symptoms. Pushed by the emotional intensity of this experience, she ventured pell-mell into the popular elaboration of midlife psychology and sociology. Summarizing her subjective experience, she wrote:

> Ireland could be explained simply. Real bullets had threatened my life from the outside. It was an observable event. My fears were appropriate. Now the destructive force was inside me. I was my own event. I could not escape it. Something alien, horrible, unspeakable, but undeniable, had begun to inhabit me. My own death. (p. 8)

This dramatic example demonstrates the connection between midlife issues and hysteria. In previous chapters, using the life cycle, we showed how the developmental approach may give new depth to

---

This chapter was written in collaboration with Robert Neborsky, M.D. The clinical examples are taken from Dr. Neborsky's work as a psychiatric consultant in a large hospital.
[1] Redesignated somatoform disorders in DSM III (1980).

the understanding and treatment of common problems in the practice of adult psychotherapy. In this chapter we begin the work that must be done to establish a comprehensive theory of midlife psychopathology by examining the relationship between adult-developmental themes and hysterical psychopathology and by demonstrating the use of these concepts in consultation and short-term work with patients.

Modern psychiatric theorists conceptualize the determinant of psychopathology in three major frameworks: the biological, the social, and the psychological. When examining any disturbed behavior—neurotic, psychotic, or characterological, the psychotherapist must parse the relative contributions of all three spheres of influence. For example, changes in bodily function in midlife can cause or precipitate psychopathology. Examples are the severe, involutional, probably biochemically mediated depressions of midlife (Rosenthal, 1968); the presenile dementias (Altzheimer's syndrome, Pick's syndrome, etc.) with destruction of brain tissue (Wells, 1971); the depressed mood and disturbed cognitive function with diminished thyroid function (Whybrow, Prange, & Treadway, 1969); and the changing hormonal levels during menopause with accompanying vasomotor instability or "hot flashes" (Reynolds, 1962). Any of these can have either primary or secondary psychological manifestations. The secondary or *somatopsychic effects* are particularly pertinent to the development of hysterical symptoms in midlife, an idea which will be expanded on later in this chapter.

Social factors that affect behavior include the family, peer group, community, and culture. Severe cultural upheavals, such as traumatic war neuroses or personality changes in concentration-camp survivors, are known to cause psychopathology in previously intact individuals. On a more subtle level, the onset of psychopathology in midlife may result from rapidly changing cultural contingencies. Since the 1960s, for example, the steady and prolonged upheaval in role expectations for women has had pervasive effects on individual lives as women have begun to assert themselves and compete with men on many levels. Social roles are in transition; many married women are now expected to assume a role identity in addition to those of spouse and mother. We observe direct relationships among these changes, the course of adult-female development, and the clinical syndrome of hysteria.

Hysterical Personality, Neurosis, and Psychosis

Nosology in Transition

Much has been written about the nosologic confusion among hysterical personality disorder, hysterical neurosis, conversion type, and somatization disorder (Briquet's syndrome). The hysterical personality disorder was initially described as a lifestyle dysfunction, the criteria for which included excitability, emotional instability, overreactivity, self-dramatization, and attention-seeking (*Diagnostic and Statistical Manual of Mental Disorders DSM* II, 1968). For complex reasons, this disorder is presently retitled histrionic personality disorder (*DSM III*, 1980). It includes no stable symptom constellations that are unpleasant or troublesome to the patient. Hysterical neurosis, conversion type, however, was, and continues to be, a specifically defined behavioral disorder in which alterations in physical functioning are present (*DSM II*, 1968; *DSM III*, 1980). Frequently the patient manifests complacency or nonchalance about the presenting symptoms (*la belle indifférence*). Psychodynamically this nonchalance is seen as the result of the denial and repression that are used to form the symptom, which usually involves impairment of the motor system (paralysis, weakness) or the sensory system (pain, anesthesia, blindness), although complex symptoms such as persistent nausea and vomiting, which have autonomic-nervous-system components, may fall under this rubric as well (Nemiah, 1975). Historically, dissociation has been seen as a possible manifestation of hysterical neurosis in amnesias and/or fugue states which function to obliterate anxiety-ridden events, memories, fantasies, or affects, but dissociation is now nosologically separate from the somatoform disorders.

Further along the continuum is hysterical psychosis (Hollender & Hirsch, 1964), which has been redesignated in *DSM III* (1980) as brief reactive psychosis—a profoundly psychotic reaction to an important dependency bond being ruptured in reality or in fantasy, with major disintegration of thinking abilities, visual and auditory hallucinations, and paranoid trends. The reaction is usually self-limited and carries no ominous prognosis of personality deterioration.

CAUSAL THEORIES AND SUBCLASSIFICATIONS

Genetic/Familial Explanations

Many authorities have heretofore been displeased with the extant methods of diagnosing hysterical disorders because of the vagueness of the criteria (Zisook, DeVaul, & Gammon, 1979). Extensive efforts to refine the inclusion criteria have led to the description of the somatization disorder or Briquet's syndrome (Guze, Woodruff, & Clayton, 1973; Perley & Guze, 1972; Purtell, Robins, & Cohen, 1951), in our opinion a positive addition to the diagnostic armamentarium. Briquet's syndrome chiefly affects women and is characterized by multiple somatic complaints that are organically unexplained. The syndrome includes varied and persistent pains, anxiety, gastrointestinal disturbances, urinary-tract malfunction, menstrual difficulties, sexual and marital maladjustment, nervousness, mood disturbances, and conversion symptoms. The course is chronic and unrelenting, including abuse of medications, frequent hospitalization, and operations. Some investigators believe it to be a *familial* condition (Arkonac & Guze, 1963) and cite a high incidence of sociopathy in first-degree male relatives (Woerner & Guze, 1968).

Psychobiological Explanation

Beginning with Charcot, Bernheim, and Janet, neurobiologists argued that conversion symptoms occur as a result of an altered state of consciousness, the hypnoid state. It was long believed that hypnotizability was an absolute requirement for the induction of hysterical symptoms. Research has disproved that assumption; hysterical patients have been shown to be no more prone to hypnosis than matched controls. However, the biological school is still strongly represented by the theories of Ludwig (1972) and Howath (Howath, Friedman, & Meares, 1980), who postulate the existence of attentional deficits along with a sham death reflex, which predisposes one to a "constant state of distraction manifest by dissociation between attention and certain sources of afferent stimulation with a simultaneous diversion of attention to non-symptom related areas" (Ludwig, 1972, p. 775).

Hysteria as an Affect Disorder

Another important somatoform, or hysterical condition, is hysterical dysphoria. Klein and Davis (1969) describe a group of patients with hysterical personalities who complain of depression, but do not manifest depressed mood in the interview situation. Those patients are reported to respond to a specific class of antidepressant medication, monoamine oxidase inhibitors. This is an important finding, but the treatment should be cautiously applied because of the potential danger of the monoamine oxidase inhibitors.

Early Psychodynamic Explanations

Ironically, the origin of psychodynamic theory and treatment was based on a largely organic conceptualization of psychopathology. Breuer and Freud (1893) were intrigued by the problem of somatic expression of emotional disorders. How, they wondered, could problems of the mind and emotions be converted into physical symptoms? Freud's early efforts were devoted to an attempt to apply electrophysiological principles to the mental apparatus. He and Breuer concluded that the pathogenic force was insufficiently discharged libido, which they conceived of as a real form of energy that demanded discharge. When counterforces of social or cultural taboos did not allow gratification of libidinal impulses, the aggregation of libido energy resulted in anxiety which was then converted into somatic symptoms (Kardiner, Karush, & Ovesey, 1959a). Freud later (1926) abandoned that conceptual model.

Modern Psychodynamic Explanations

The adult cognition of the hysterical patient has been exquisitely described by Shapiro (1965) and later by Horowitz (1972, 1977). In short, hysterical individuals tend to minimize or deny the implications of external events and repress unacceptable thoughts, fantasies, and affects. The emergence of powerful midlife developmental themes and conflicts may disturb the precarious intrapsychic balance found in many such people and precipitate symptom formation, often through the use of conversion mechanisms. In an extensive review, Rangell (1959) emphasizes the importance of conversion as a psychodynamic *process* which the ego invokes when confronted with conflict between the infantile determinants and the adaptive context.

Marmor (1953), Easser and Lesser (1965), Zetzel (1968), and Kernberg (1976) among others, have cited early-oral-stage developmental fixations, and/or arrests and deviations, as the predisposing factor in the vulnerabilities of hysterical personalities. Following Freud, Reich (1933/1969) and again Zetzel (1965) have described the continuing unresolved oedipal conflicts which are central in the formation of hysterical symptoms and character structures.

Sociocultural Explanations

Social factors are often overlooked as determinants in the production of hysterical psychopathology, and evidence in the literature is sparse except in cross-cultural studies. There are those, however, who suggest that hysterical psychopathology is an expression of psychosocial stress resulting from cultural change (Temoshok & Attkisson, 1977). Halleck (1967) relates the development of hysteria to the tendency in American society to encourage aggression and suppress dependency needs in males, while fostering highly dependent roles in women. Supporting that view, Hollender (1980) reexamines the famous case of Anna O., stressing the sociocultural determinants of her psychopathology and the relationship of those factors to the birth of dynamic psychotherapy.

CLINICAL APPLICATIONS

The core hypothesis of this chapter is that midlife developmental pressures can strongly influence the onset and course of hysterical symptoms. During the middle years people experience a need to act when confronted unequivocally with the finitude of their existence. The style of one's cognition dictates whether that experience occurs consciously or unconsciously, and, by definition, hysterical character defenses push ego-dystonic thoughts out of consciousness.

For some, midlife provides another chance, or perhaps the final chance. Many women experience a new freedom when relieved of responsibilities for child care. Careers once postponed can now be engaged. Often, though, rationalizations for inactivity which have protected the ego from a loss of self-esteem are dissolved by reality, and midlife itself results in a new stress, upsetting character defenses and necessitating more neurotic defensive operations.

Middle-aged individuals with hysterical tendencies often use their bodies to express their neurotic conflicts. The development of the motor system, for example, is intimately related to the separation-individuation process and patients may manifest conflicts along that developmental line, their conversion symptoms symbolically expressing the inability to move forward. To demonstrate these and other concepts we have chosen four patients seen in brief treatment in whom the midlife psychological factors are particularly apparent. From medical and psychiatric standpoints all four cases were complex. A preoccupation with physical well-being existed in each patient, necessitating thorough medical, neurological, and endocrinological evaluations which failed to demonstrate causative organic pathology. In each case the attending physician worked in close collaboration with the consulting psychiatrist.

Clinical Vignettes

"Last Chance": The Emergence of the Wish to Be First

A. was a conspicuously attractive 49-year-old woman who appeared for psychiatric consultation after an extensive medical workup for a choreaform tremor in her right hand (writer's cramp). The tremor totally interfered with her ability to write, especially checks. Two years earlier she had experienced an episode of paralytic Guillain-Barré syndrome which remitted with steroid therapy after an eight-month course. The onset of her tremor coincided with consideration of her husband for an important executive position in a multinational conglomerate which would require an extended overseas stay. A. had strong negative feelings about the move, whereas her husband looked forward to it with relish. She sought aid from a female hypnotherapist, but hypnosis failed to produce symptomatic relief. A. became particularly anxious at corporate social gatherings and developed incipient agoraphobia on the way to those functions.

The eldest daughter of a middle-class, midwestern family, she fondly recalled her father who, despite limited formal education, was a good provider and a respected member of their community. Childhood was glowingly happy, with no unpleasant experiences. Always an achiever, A. described her past as nice, happy, average, and so on. After graduation from college she began a career but abandoned it to marry

M., an exciting, handsome, understanding, and effective man. They so-journed through a military commitment in which M. distinguished him-self in combat. Two daughters were born during the military tenure, and later a son when A. was 36. All three children developed normally.

During A.'s evaluation the promotion was confirmed. WAIS, MMPI, and Rorschach tests were interpreted as compatible with a conversion re-action in a hysterical, neurotic character structure: "In large part, her motor tremulousness can be seen as an unconscious representation of her *trembling* with rage, in a woman who has sought to model herself along lines of being proper, dutiful and controlled, a woman who funda-mentally believes that feeling and acting angrily and forcefully asserting her own interest would be "not to act like a woman" . . . a woman who feels tremendous guilt as she becomes angry; yet a woman who is strug-gling with the feeling that she has subordinated her wishes to those of the family for too long and who now is experiencing the prohibited but conflicted wish that her husband would care enough about her to put her wishes above all else . . . ."

A. agreed to participate in four months of intensive psychodynamic psychotherapy during which time she would decide whether or not to accompany her husband. She quickly assumed a dependent, angry pos-ture; she felt frustrated by the therapist's lack of direction, and the ab-sence of concrete "help." Despite the frustration A. maintained a viable therapeutic alliance, and after the first month of treatment began report-ing dreams. "M. and I have two children. We are not married. He's off with another woman. I felt like there must be some way to explain to him that we need him [slip: you]. I loved him and missed him. Somehow at the end we were together. He's saying, 'It's all right. I understand.' "

To our line of reasoning, this dream reflected both adult-developmental and infantile conflicts. From the adult-developmental point of view, midlife offered A. her "last chance" for individuation and increased self-esteem, "to be my own person, not just his wife." M.'s leaving with another woman (his career) created intense anxiety and an-ger. A.'s life had been built around being a mother and dutiful wife. Now the children were gone, and her husband was asking for a major sacrifice. In the dream she rebels and strikes out on her own, only to ex-perience loneliness and a desire for rapprochement and forgiveness. The therapist, perhaps as indicated by the slip, is a transitional object to help conquer the anticipated loneliness should she choose to remain behind. Understood in oedipal terms, the dream represented the conflict be-tween her love for her husband/father and her rage because he chose an-other (career/mother).

A crisis occurred when A.'s anxiety outpaced the growth of the ther-apeutic alliance and she felt compelled to terminate treatment because of the lack of "help" from the therapist. After consulting a psychologist friend, she returned to treatment (without missing a session) with new commitment and entered the middle phase of her therapy, in which strong depressive feelings emerged. The mental content of the depressed mood was grief over the loss of the intimacy she experienced with her fa-ther. Always efficient and dutiful, A. had organized his funeral when he died shortly after her graduation from college. She was unable to grieve until the therapeutic process released those feelings.

Her tremor had not changed; if anything, it had increased in severity and frequency, so that two months into treatment, imipramine, 150 mg at bedtime, was prescribed. A.'s mood and agoraphobia improved with three weeks of imipramine treatment and continued ventilation of her grief over her father's death and rage at her husband's seeming neglect. Her dream material shifted to themes of being single and wandering in the Orient, walking down streets and viewing magical knobs and buttons that "tell you the height of tidal waves in Japan." She continued to work on the conflict between her own needs and wishes and the duty and responsibility she felt toward her children and husband. The transference gradually changed to a strongly positive one with deeply felt gratitude and feelings of intimacy. The erotic components of the transference were in the main repressed and not dealt with since symptomatic relief was obtained at that point without symbolic interpretation. Two weeks prior to termination A. decided to go with M., but vowed to pursue her own interests and career while there. Arrangements were made for psychiatric follow-up. After two weeks of work on separation from the therapist, her therapy ended on a markedly positive note.

Midlife Stagnation, Precipitated by the Need to Be a Child Again

B. was a 48-year-old, married woman referred for evaluation of the persistent sensation of a lump in her throat (globus hystericus), headaches, and dizziness. Her symptoms had begun five years earlier and were associated with insomnia. The precipitant was the separation from home of her eldest daughter and soon thereafter a second child as well. B. felt a vacuum in her life and began a second career as a personnel counselor for a moderate-sized corporation. At that time she began medicating herself with Dalmane, Phenergan, and Benadryl. After perceiving herself as depressed and seeking psychiatric help, she was placed on Elavil, which seemed to relieve her symptoms but was discontinued after she experienced terrifying visual hallucinations of "large black objects" coming at her. Thereafter the globus hystericus developed, and B. admitted herself to a clinic for a check of "hormonal balance." Just prior to referral she had received an extensive medical workup which failed to reveal any endocrinologic etiology for the symptoms.

B. was the eldest daughter among five siblings; one brother was five years older than she; two sisters and one brother were younger. The early family history was marked by much trauma and disruption. Both parents were severe alcoholics. B. was raised in a small midwestern town where "everyone knew everyone else." Her father, it seems, was an episodic drinker who became extremely violent during his binges, beating older brother and mother but avoiding the female children. Mother also drank to the point of unconsciousness, causing B. much shame and embarrassment. She recalled feeling terror at father's threats to interrupt her education, a source of great self-esteem. In the eighth grade she avoided home by working excessively long hours in part-time jobs.

Father developed a tyrannical attitude toward her dating while mother began using B. as a confidante, discussing her husband's erotic behavior and frequent infidelity. When B. was 18, father died from cancer, producing a feeling of great relief, as if "justice had been done." B.'s first experience with insomnia occurred during his fatal illness.

After his death she moved to the West Coast and became quite successful as a fashion merchandiser. Many offers of marriage followed, all refused on the grounds that none of the men was "good enough." B. feared that she was "uncontrollable," and selected a husband with a very strong personality who was warm and giving as well. Her one mission was to provide well for her children, to make certain they never experienced the deprivation she had known. After the birth of their second child, B. and her husband decided to have no more children, and soon thereafter she experienced severe sexual problems. Despite an interest in sex, she began refusing her husband's advances.

Therapy was intended to "prime the pump" for extended, intensive psychotherapy closer to home. Consultation revealed marked use of denial, repression, and somatization to deal with conflicts representing underlying narcissistic disturbances. The headaches and dizziness seemed to be related to separation conflicts precipitated by children leaving home. B. had maintained her equilibrium by adopting the role of "supermom" in a magical attempt to repair the deprivation experienced as a child. When that adaptation was shattered by the development of her children, she underwent hypochondriacal regression, abandoned the sexual relationship with her husband, and became the child who needed to be cared for by him, the good parent. B.'s earlier sublimatory outlet as a fashion merchandiser could not be regained because of the regression, and she remained fixed in psychosomatic symptomatology. The infantile conflicts represented by the globus hystericus were not determined in the relatively brief evaluation.

Obviously, not all of B.'s psychopathology could be ascribed to midlife conflicts, but her case does highlight the intertwining of the adaptive tasks of midlife with underlying developmental fixation. B. suffered much deprivation as a young child, for neither parent was emotionally available to her. Although deeply scarred, she was able to separate from the situation and succeed as a fashion merchandiser, a career related to the material deprivation of her earlier years. One of her most traumatic memories was the shame and embarrassment she experienced wearing underwear made of burlap flour sacks to school. Midlife was a time when the traumata and conflicts of childhood returned. No longer could she fend off depression and anger by being a "superwoman," married to a "superhusband." Without the children, B. had to deal with the reemergence of a powerful need to be a helpless child, continually cared for by an attentive parent.

"Time's Winged Chariot": The Inability to Recapture the Lost Father

C. was a 48-year-old woman writer who had undergone extensive medical evaluation for periodic falling spells (abasia), anxiety, and uncontrollable coughing (tussis nervosa). Her symptom of falling and fainting was so disabling that she had collapsed at a public concert. About six months before the consultation she had resigned a position as a newspaper columnist to pursue a lifelong wish to be a novelist. C. had been engaged in extensive research for the book and had divorced herself from many social contacts, "unaware" of any stress in her life.

An only child, C. was born when father was in his late thirties and mother in her late twenties. Both parents wished for more children, but mother suffered three miscarriages after C. was born. C. described herself as a bright and precocious child who was "too pretty for her own good." When asked to explain that statement, she related the suffering caused by the jealousy of her classmates and their parents which eventually lead to a change of school.

C.'s relationship with her father, a genius who built a small neighborhood newspaper into a large urban newspaper, was conflicted. She remembered parental bickering over "too much newspaper" and not enough family. At age 16 she eloped against her parent's wishes; the marriage was subsequently annulled. Three years later she remarried, and her only child was born. Divorce soon followed. C. remarked spontaneously that with men she had always felt continual disappointment, because of her expectation of perfection. Since the last marriage ended she had not established another long-term relationship. Now time was running out. Three years before her consultation, C.'s father died suddenly of a heart attack; two weeks before that he had left C.'s mother to live with a younger woman. C. recalled grieving heavily when he died.

Therapy with this woman was brief and directed at creating a positive attitude, setting the stage for treatment in another city. Initially she worked on anger about her lot in midlife. C. had always felt herself to be the source of envy for other women; this attitude was the fountainhead of her self-esteem. Now the tables were turned. She was envious of women who "captured" men as their spouses. She began to work through feelings of rage at her father for his unconventional behavior (an elaborate rationalization for her oedipal jealousy over his rejection of her?) and came to grips with strong feelings of loneliness and isolation. At last report she remained in intensive psychotherapy in her home city and, after one exacerbation, was asymptomatic.

"The May-December Ritual": A Repetitive Compulsion

D., a 40-year-old woman, was referred for consultation after a year of episodic nausea and vomiting without apparent medical cause. In that year she was hospitalized four times for management of the resulting dehydration. D. could identify no situational factors, but did admit to occasional "nervousness." Her attitude was one of indifference, and she seemed irritated when the interviewer probed beneath the surface.

The sequence of events was invariable. D. would eat, experience mild abdominal distension, panic, feel a lump in her throat, then begin vomiting with intractable retching. She was not abusing alcohol, despite a history of episodic "alcoholism" in the past. The patient was living with a sailor 20 years her junior, after leaving the last of seven husbands (all sailors) in order to marry this young man. There were "no problems in the relationship," despite the presence at home of three children, one the age of her lover.

D. was the illegitimate child of a sailor, a man she never met. She disliked both her mother and stepfather and experienced little or no closeness with either of them, in part because their relationship was one of constant bickering and frequent physical fighting. At age 15 D. ran away from home, became promiscuous, and was involved "with a gang of rough blacks." Against her will she was placed in a reform school where for the next three years she was forced to participate in homosexual activities.

The diagnostic impression was severe hysterical neurosis (Briquet's syndrome) with an underlying borderline character structure. In close collaboration with the patient's gastroenterologist, treatment involved supportive psychotherapy and low doses of antianxiety medication to diminish the episodic vomiting. It was apparent that D. was terrified of getting older and losing her attractiveness to men. Each of her seven husbands had been younger than his predecessor. Her hopeless compulsion to marry progressively younger sailors/fathers confirmed that the infantile trauma caused by an absent, idealized father had never been mastered. The patient did not return for psychotherapy after the initial evaluation.

Two months later she was in the hospital, grossly psychotic, running up and down the halls of the medical wards, screaming and actively hallucinating. Emergency sedation was ordered and in a few days it was possible to reconstruct the recent history. D. had returned to drinking and was at her local tavern where she met her lover's best friend (also a sailor) and acceded to his sexual advances. The next day she felt intense shame and began to vomit. An emergency-room diagnosis of acute cholecystitis led to admission. On the way to the ward D. fantasized that her lover would leave her because of the affair and experienced visual hallucinations of the primal scene—a sailor making love to a woman. Next she envisioned a fight between her two lovers, and believed she was dead, wrapped in a cheesecloth shroud. A few days later, no longer psychotic, D. was discharged and recognized the need for further therapy. She was able to accept a supportive relationship and verbalize her fears of abandonment in midlife. Soon after her oldest son left home, and she married her lover, who never discovered the affair. There have been no episodes of vomiting since therapy resumed, likely because of the support and acceptance of the therapist, a younger man.

THERAPEUTIC ALLIANCE AND EXPLORATION OF THE SELF

In many ways the clinician has the deck stacked against him in the treatment of hysterical disorders (Fairbarn, 1954). The combination of denial, repression, and somatization militates against therapeutic leverage. However, the psychosocial situation of the midlife dilemma is an issue that patients readily comprehend, providing a comfortable framework within which to build an alliance. In fact, at the onset of an evaluation patients often spontaneously refer to their "midlife crisis." Resistance usually appears when the therapist tries to explore the relationship between the childhood developmental past and the adult present either prematurely or with patients who are not psychologically minded. At times pharmacological intervention will help consolidate a shaky therapeutic alliance by providing immediate relief and a sense that the therapist actively cares.

TRANSFERENCE MANIFESTATIONS AND MIDLIFE ISSUES

In each of the above cases, the psychiatrist, a male, was younger than the woman in treatment. This issue was of great psychodynamic importance to patient A., who often wondered aloud if the therapist had the years "to understand what she was going through." In our terms, she was asking about his capacity for developmental resonance. Without active assistance from the therapist, many patients are unable to verbalize thoughts that they feel are "inappropriate" to the age differences involved.

> Mrs. S., age 45, divorced for many years and now a successful realtor, came to treatment because of continued anger over her 20-year-old son, who had just "come out" as a homosexual and was living with a man years older than he. A therapeutic alliance developed fairly quickly, but the material was dry and intellectual. Eventually, confronted with her fear of expressing emotions to a younger therapist, the patient responded that she was sexually aroused by the therapist, but afraid to discuss those feelings. When the feelings were explored, she came to understand that the source of her fury toward her son's lover (to whom she was sexually attracted), was his having chosen her son over her.

COUNTERTRANSFERENCE

There are at least three distinct influences on the countertransference manifestations presented by midlife patients with psychopathology amenable to dynamic treatment. One aspect is the general countertransference experienced with hysterical patients. The second is the general countertransference affects experienced in dealing with midlife psychology. The third is the specific problems of a younger therapist dealing with transferences of midlife patients of the opposite sex. That aspect will be the focus of this section of the discussion.

An implicit paradox exists in the transference relationship with a youthful therapist. Traditionally, the idealized psychotherapist is seen as older, wiser, a more experienced help-giver for the patient. The reality of the therapist's youth contradicts this expectation and creates a role reversal with which the therapist must deal. Once that is done, the traditional transference phenomena begin to emerge, largely along classical lines. However, the adult-developmental transference material continues to be influenced by the age disparity since the therapist represents a constant reminder of two central midlife issues: loss of the youthful body (aging), and the finiteness of time (loss of omnipotentiality). For this reason the therapist's presence itself, no matter how well intentioned, can be the source of a narcissistic injury, against which the patient must defend. This is a very difficult technical area of therapy, because the therapist himself has not yet weathered this specific developmental phase, and empathic resonance may be impaired. It cannot be overemphasized how aware the therapist must be of this aspect of his relatedness to the patient. The resolution of this issue often revolves around the recognition that the patient has unique cognitive and emotional perspectives on life from which the therapist can learn.

Finally, the younger therapist finds himself dealing with intense countertransference feelings toward patients who may represent aspects of his own parents. If these paradigms go unrecognized, empathic dissonance can result. These anxieties are usually specific to the psychodynamics of the therapist, and may appear along any of the developmental lines. One area of particular sensitivity is the recapitulation of oedipal conflicts, since the representation of the therapist as a youthful child-lover may stir up unresolved oedipal conflicts in the therapist.

RECONSTRUCTION: SYMBOLIC FUNCTION OF SYMPTOMS

We feel special emphasis should be placed on the issue of aging and changes in the adult body in relation to hysterical psychopathology at midlife. It is our conviction that aging changes in the adult body are reflected in mental representations, and according to that principle, each of the four patients discussed above communicated symbolically through motor symptoms a perception of her midlife dilemma: A. trembled with rage and fear, caught between dutiful loyalty to her husband and impulses to flee and pay (with checks) her *own* way in the world. B., fatigued, depressed, and sexually withdrawn from her husband, was unable to swallow without a lump in her throat. In addition to the traditional oral-phallic interpretations, one wonders if her symptom also symbolized the *stagnation* experienced when the caregiver role was lost and she was forced to move to a less symbiotic source of gratification. C.'s abasia may have represented her perception of an inability to stand on her own feet without male support while her friends had husbands. D.'s nausea and vomiting may have reflected her impaired ability to trust the adult world for support. She compulsively and repetitively remarried and seduced men in attempts to recapture the basic trust she never internalized due to her early years of deprivation.

Successful short-term psychotherapy or crisis intervention does not depend on such reconstructions being made; in fact, none was with these particular patients. The goal was not necessarily insight into unconscious infantile motivations, but the ability to proceed with adult-developmental themes without pronounced regression or fixation.

REFERENCES

Arkonac, O., & Guze, S. A family study of hysteria. *New England Journal of Medicine*, 1963, *268*, 239.

Breuer, J., & Freud, S. *On the psychical mechanisms of hysterical phenomena.* Standard edition, 2:1. London: Hogarth Press, 1893.

Diagnostic and Statistical Manual of Mental Disorders II. Washington, D.C.: American Psychiatric Association, 1968.

Diagnostic and Statistical Manual of Mental Disorders III. Washington, D.C.: American Psychiatric Association, 1980.

Easser, B. R., & Lesser, S. R. Hysterical personality: A revaluation. *Psychoanalytic Quarterly*, 1965, *34*, 390.

Fairbarn, W. R. Observations on the nature of hysterical states. *British Journal of Medical Psychology*, 1954, *27*, 105.

Freud, S. *Inhibitions, symptoms, and anxiety*. Standard edition, 20:177. London: Hogarth Press, 1926.

Guze, S. B., Woodruff, R. A., & Clayton, P. A. Sex, age and the diagnosis of hysteria (Briquet's syndrome). *American Journal of Psychiatry*, 1973, *129*, 745.

Halleck, S. L. Hysterical personality: Psychological, social, and iatrogenic determinants. *Archives of General Psychiatry*, 1967, *16*, 750.

Hollender, M. H. The case of Anna O.: A reformulation. *American Journal of Psychiatry*, 1980, *137*, 797.

Hollender, M. H., & Hirsch, W. J. Hysterical psychosis. *American Journal of Psychiatry*, 1964, *120*, 1066.

Horowitz, M. Modes of representation of thought. *Journal of the American Psychoanalytic Association*, 1972, *20*, 793.

Horowitz, M. (Ed.). *Hysterical personality*. New York: Jason Aronson, 1977.

Horvath, T., Friedman, J., & Meares, R. Attention in hysteria: A study of Janet's hypothesis by means of habituation and arousal measures. *American Journal of Psychiatry*, 1980, *137*, 217.

Kardiner, A., Karush, A., & Ovesey, L. A methodological study of Freudian theory, II. The libido theory. *Journal of Nervous and Mental Disorder*, 1959, *129*, 133. (a)

Kardiner, A., Karush, A., & Ovesey, L. A methodological study of Freudian theory, IV. The structural hypotheses, the problem of anxiety, and post-Freudian ego psychology. *Journal of Nervous and Mental Disorder*, 1959, *129*, 341. (b)

Kernberg, O. *Object relations theory and clinical psychoanalysis*. New York: Jason Aronson, 1976.

Klein, D. F., & Davis, J. M. *Diagnosis and drug treatment of psychiatric disorders*. Baltimore: Waverly, 1969.

Ludwig, A. M. Hysteria: A neurobiologic theory. *Archives of General Psychiatry*, 1972, *27*, 771.

Marmor, J. Orality in the hysterical personality. *Journal of the American Psychoanalytic Association*, 1953, *1*, 656.

Nemiah, J. Hysterical neurosis, conversion type. In A. Freedman & H. Kaplan (Eds.), *Comprehensive textbook of psychiatry I*. Baltimore: William & Wilkins, 1975, pp. 1208–1220.

Perley, T. M., & Guze, S. B. Hysteria: The stability and usefulness of clinical criteria. *New England Journal of Medicine*, 1972, *266*, 421.

Purtell, J. J., Robins, E., & Cohen, M. E. Observations on clinical aspects of hysteria: A quantitative study of fifty patients and one hundred fifty six control subjects. *Journal of the American Medical Association*, 1951, *146*, 902.

Rangell, L. The nature of conversion. *Journal of the American Psychoanalytic Association*, 1959, *17*, 632.

Reich, W. *Character analysis*. New York: Farrar, Straus, & Giroux, 1969. (Originally published, 1933.)

Reynolds, S. Physiological and psychogenic factors in the menopausal flush syndrome. In W. Kroger (Ed.), *Psychosomatic obstetrics, gynecology, and endocrinology*. Springfield, Ill.: Charles C Thomas, 1962.

Rosenthal, S. H. The involutional depressive syndrome. *American Journal of Psychiatry*, 1968, *124* (Suppl. 21).

Shapiro, D. *Neurotic styles*. New York: Basic Books, 1965.

Sheehy, G. *Passages*. New York: E. P. Dutton, 1974.

Temoshok, L., & Attkisson, C. C. Epidemiology of hysterical phenomena: Evidence for a psychosocial theory. In M. Horowitz (Ed.), *Hysterical personality*. New York: Aronson, 1977, pp. 146-222.

Wells, C. E. *Dementia*. Philadelphia: F. A. Davis, 1971.

Whybrow, P. C., Prange, A. J., & Treadway, C. R. Mental changes accompanying thyroid gland dysfunction. *Archives of General Psychiatry*, 1969, *20*, 48.

Woerner, P. J., & Guze, S. B. A family and mental study of hysteria. *British Journal of Psychiatry*, 1968, *114*, 161.

Zetzel, E. The so-called good hysteric. *International Journal of Psycho-Analysis*, 1968, *48*, 256.

Zisook, S., DeVaul, R. A., & Gammon, E. The hysterical facade. *American Journal of Psychoanalysis*, 1979, *39*, 113.

15

Adult Development and the Educational Process

The implications of the developmental orientation for the educational process are myriad, affecting what is taught, how it is communicated, and the roles of students and teachers. Although we speak specifically about the educational process as it relates to the mental-health professions, many of the developmental concepts presented are applicable to any learning situation since experiences as student and teacher are an integral part of the human condition.

This chapter is divided into four parts. The first section describes the basic educational objectives to be achieved in teaching developmental theory to mental-health students. The second section focuses on the developmental experiences of the students, the third explores the complex, interlocking relationship between student-therapist and supervisor. The last section is devoted to sample courses on development and student reaction to them.

OBJECTIVES

To Present the Normal Developmental Theory of the Life Cycle

The student should study the *entire* life cycle, from infancy to old age, since all phases of development are interconnected and each succeeding phase builds upon previous ones. Normal developmental theory should be taught formally and informally throughout the training period.

Theoretical concepts should be brought to life by the *direct observa-*

tion of children, adults, and families. These observations should be *serial*, covering all phases of development from infancy to old age; and *longitudinal*, for example, observing an individual mother–child dyad or family throughout the training period.

To Relate Developmental Concepts to Psychopathology, Diagnosis, and Treatment

The major psychopathological processes of childhood and adulthood should be formally presented and illustrated through case presentations and interviews to help the student understand the *correlation* between adult psychopathology and childhood developmental processes and problems. As these ideas are related to the growing fund of knowledge about normal development (which is taught concurrently), the student begins to define the similarities and differences between normal and pathological processes at various stages of the life cycle.

Diagnostic techniques should be taught that place developmental concepts and the developmental history of the life cycle—not just childhood—in the center of the diagnostic process. Differences in diagnostic techniques that are dictated by developmental concepts, such as the involvement of parents in the evaluation of children, should be illustrated. Students should observe and conduct diagnostic evaluations on individuals of all ages.

Students should come to recognize that psychotherapeutic technique is determined in part by the stage of development of the patient and in part by his level of progression upon individual developmental lines. Furthermore, the interaction between therapist and patient is strongly influenced by their relative positions in the life cycle. Of paramount significance is the recognition that the goal of treatment is the assumption of normal developmental processes rather than only symptom removal.

In order to integrate these concepts each student should have experience in treating, under supervision, individuals of all ages. The *effect* of therapeutic intervention on the freeing up of developmental processes should be illustrated in continual case conferences and experienced through the long-term treatment of patients.

To Utilize Developmental Concepts in Curriculum Planning and Teaching

As suggested in the Conference on Psychoanalytic Education and Research, Commission IX report (1974), a "spiral curriculum" model should be utilized. Basic concepts are introduced and then repeated and elaborated upon throughout the training years by connecting them to other ideas and aspects of training. For example, normal developmental concepts are first presented as a framework from which to understand human behavior and then related to psychopathology and psychotherapy. Use of this model presupposes the student as a dynamic, evolving person capable of more complex integration as the training period progresses.

Whenever possible, courses should be taught jointly by male and female instructors who have between them experience with both adults and children.

Supervision is a complex developmental interaction between supervisor and supervisee. The supervisor should be cognizant of the fact that it is not only the student who is changed and influenced by their interaction, but himself as well.

To Encourage Research and Writing about Developmental Concepts

The opportunities for clinical or laboratory research on development are multiple during the training years. The emergence of the capacity for writing and research is a developmental task that can be either ignored or stimulated during the training years. Each training program should actively provide time, direction, and mentors to facilitate the emergence of this vital aspect of professional identity.

To Further the Developmental Potential of Each Student to Its Fullest

It is the obligation of every teacher, based on deep respect for the individual student, to structure the training program in such a way as to promote the *total* development of each trainee. Training demands should be kept at a reasonable level to allow time and energy for young families and other interests. The capacity of the faculty to resonate with the developmental demands of the young-adult student will determine the appropriateness of all training expectations.

Educational Developmental Sequences in the Student

The education of psychiatrists and other mental-health workers is a developmental experience that is an integral part of the ongoing development of early adulthood. When understood and utilized by students and teachers, this fact can have a major effect on the educational process. Knowledge of the details involved is still rudimentary, but it is growing. In this section, relying on the seminal ideas contained in the Commission IX report (1974) and in those few articles that have approached mental-health education from a developmental standpoint, we will address some of the important developmental issues that affect mental-health training.

Candidate Selection and Progression

The developmental orientation can be extremely halpful in *candidate selection* since it provides a perspective from which to assess suitability for training. Particular attention can be paid to those developmental lines that lead to the emergence of object relatedness and the capacities for sensitivity and empathy—prerequisites for psychotherapeutic work with patients. By studying the developmental line of work identity, the decision to become a mental-health professional can be traced to its origins, often in late adolescence, and a determination made of the validity of such a decision in light of *current* developmental objectives. All of this information can be placed in the broader framework of degree of emotional intactness and stability, the ultimate determinants of suitability for training, through a thorough investigation of the individual's experiences in the life cycle, from infancy through the present.

If the student is understood to be a developing individual, it will be recognized that *progression itself is a developmental process* that occurs at highly individual rates and is subject to regression and fixation. An attempt should be made to understand the mode and sequence of learning employed by each student and to tailor educational demands and expectations to the individual. A rigid curriculum that demands that every student learn the same material at the same rate of speed is just as inappropriate at a postgraduate level as it is in elementary school. Furthermore, allowances need to be made for individual experience with current adult-developmental tasks that affect and interdigitate with training demands.

The Dilemma of the Adult Student

No matter how sensitive the educator may be, nothing can prevent the divergent effects and influences that graduate and postgraduate education have on other adult-developmental tasks. In his 1969 Presidential Address to the American Psychoanalytic Association, Samuel Ritvo (1971) spoke sensitively of this developmental dilemma of the psychoanalytic candidate. His words are just as valid for other students.

> Contemporary society requires an increasingly prolonged student status as young adults pursue graduate education. This prolongation is difficult enough in the twenties, but it runs counter to the natural stream and rhythm of life when it extends into the thirties and forties as it does for analytic candidates and many graduate students. The combined regressive pull of the training analysis and the continuation of student status when life tasks are, in Erikson's terms, in the generative phase, greatly tax the candidate's strength and maturity. In addition, the financial and temporal demands of being in a student situation that goes counter to the normal course of training conflict with the candidate's desire and obligation to meet the needs of a wife and young children, which are at a peak at this time. The result is the all-too-familiar picture of tired students crowding a central life interest into evenings, weekends, or odd hours during the day. (p. 14)

Pregnancy, Motherhood, and Training

The education and training of psychiatric residents, psychologists, and social workers should be organized so as to promote *total* adult development. Since the emergence of a professional work identity is a major developmental task of young adulthood, personal and professional development *merge* in the training experience and are in part synonymous.

This important concept is illustrated by our experience with four female psychiatric residents, all trying to mesh their desire for motherhood with their training. In each instance, we as educators explored the questions brought to us by these residents, using as our primary frame of reference their total development as adults.

One woman in her middle thirties, contemplating pregnancy, inquired about the effects of delaying her child-psychiatry training in order to have a child. She was encouraged to delay her training and pursue her wish to become a mother. Her age dictated that the ability to produce a healthy child was time-limited, whereas the option for training would remain open in the future. Furthermore, becoming a parent would add an important dimension to her training experience.

A second woman, seven months pregnant, was amazed at the powerful effect of her pregnancy on herself and her patients. Being a pregnant therapist provided her with a unique opportunity to observe the intense sexual response produced in a male-adolescent patient and the envy aroused in a female patient of childbearing age. But most impressive was her own increased preoccupation with her body and the baby inside. Gradually she began to experience psychotherapeutic involvement with patients as an *intrusion* into a normal, growing psychological preoccupation with her body. An empathic discussion of these feelings helped the resident define the limits of her willingness to meet the needs of others when they conflicted with her own. Instead of working until the last month of the pregnancy as originally planned, she decided to stop sooner to allow more time and energy to explore her own physical and psychological response to the individual growing inside of her.

A third woman, who delivered during the third year of residency and was the mother of a three-month-old, was amazed at the power of her investment in her child. She had read about the early mother–child relationship, but now she was living it. After considerable discussion she decided to postpone child-psychiatry training for a year or two in order to fully engage the developmental experience of motherhood. "It will be a learning experience, too," she added. "I know the theory. Now I'm going to test it out firsthand."

A fourth woman, the mother of two, asked to take her residency training on a part-time basis to allow her to balance the twin adult tasks of motherhood and professional development. An individual program was tailored for her to facilitate achievement of these legitimate developmental goals.

The Future Teacher

The future teacher is emerging even as the beginning student is learning. Through identifications and opportunities to teach and supervise, knowledge is integrated and professional identity is solidified. This developmental process, which is phase-specific for the training period, should be conceptualized as an integral part of the training experience and formally built into the program. Early and progressive acknowledgement of future roles as teacher and administrator as well as therapist should be a component of assessment and feedback during the training years. An illustration of this necessity was experienced in the University of California Psychiatric Residency Program. In the early years of the program the entire third year of the residency was conceived of as elective time. When this policy was studied by the faculty, it was found that only a few residents were really able to utilize that year effectively. Subsequently, a final year was constructed that included opportunities for residents to have senior- and chief-resident responsibilities, continued clinical work, and elective research opportunities. The changes facilitated *the transition to the teacher role as an essential part of the training experience.* After some resistance to change, the third and final year of the residency program, with its emphasis on a developmental integration of tasks and skills from previous years, was described by many students as the "single most meaningful experience in the entire program."

Graduation indicates the arrival at yet another stage on the developmental continuum. Experiences during the training years and in the years thereafter complement and interact in the continuing evolution of professional identity and activity. Thus, the therapist's evolution is powerfully affected by new adult experiences, such as marriage, parenthood, and so forth, which change the individual and alter his or her perspectives on patients, work, and his or her own self. And within the training continuum the evolution continues as the new teacher engages the new student, as illustrated by the supervisor–supervisee interaction.

PSYCHOTHERAPY: THE DEVELOPMENTAL CRUCIBLE FOR STUDENT AND
SUPERVISOR

There are enormous anxieties involved in becoming a psychotherapist. They grow out of the need to forge a therapeutic identity, a
process that takes many years. "The beginner often denies this. He
may have to if he is to retain his self-esteem among unfamiliar persons
and challenges" (Van Buskirk, 1969, p. 46).

The unfamiliar persons are patients and supervisors, and the challenges are multiple. Among them are the necessity to "understand em-
pathically; structure relationships cooperatively; use himself as the instrument of observation and treatment and tolerate psychic conflict"
(Van Buskirk, 1969, p. 52).

During the initial year of training, a psychiatric resident is plunged
into a morass of newness. Asked to disregard the classical medical approach toward therapy and disease, and estranged to some degree
from his former colleagues, he must surrender a new and often painfully acquired identity. The doctor–patient relationship must be redefined. An awareness of ancillary services as more than mere medical
adjuncts must be fostered. Moreover, it is necessary to come to grips
with the reality that nurses, aides, social workers, and occupational
and physical therapists are often more adept at handling disturbed behavior. In essence, a beginning resident is confronted with an enormous challenge to his self-esteem at a time when he is struggling to establish a new professional identity.

The feelings of inexperience and relative helplessness in the new
role of therapist stand in sharp contrast to the relative comfort achieved
outside of the training situation in regard to such developmental tasks
as intimacy, marriage, and parenthood. The experience of being an accomplished adult stands in juxtaposition to the anxiety that is generated by therapy sessions. Becoming a therapist is not analogous to acquiring just another skill because, as previously described, the
therapist must use *himself* as the instrument of observation and treatment. The involvement of the self in such a process stresses the current
intrapsychic equilibrium but at the same time serves as a vehicle to *future* emotional development in a manner that is unrealized in other
adult work activities.

The Apprentice Complex

The initial inexperience and anxiety generated by psychotherapy bring us to the supervisory experience, the crucible in which the identity of therapist—and supervisor—is forged. In an attempt to cope with the demands of the therapeutic situation the student may develop what Ornstein (1968) calls the "apprentice complex." The beginning therapist approaches his supervisor feeling like the sorcerer's apprentice. That poor student, possessing no magic of his own, stole his master's magic, only to discover that it was something he could not control.

> The teacher is put on the pedestal, admired, imitated and seen as possessing all the answers the trainee is looking for, as being the ultimate authority to whom the resident defers in all professional matters . . . . This kind of excessive deference, or its opposite hidden or overt, interferes with the trainee's genuine reflective presence in the relationship with his patient. (p. 301)

What Ornstein is describing, we believe, is the initial phase in the relationship of mentee to mentor, therapist to supervisor. The idealization described is, we believe, an integral part of the process of engaging the mentor and therefore potentially positive and growth promoting.

A Preceptorship for Beginning Psychiatric Residents

In the following paragraphs we shall describe a unique mentor-supervisory experience (Nemiroff & Tischler, 1977) which had particular developmental relevance for beginning psychiatric residents. We believe the model of a preceptorship, which has considerable training potential, has been underutilized. Between 1963 and 1966, the Department of Psychiatry of Yale University provided a group of 12 first-year residents with a newly conceived learning experience entitled "An Experiment in Self-Exploration." Each resident had an opportunity to meet privately with a training analyst from the Western New England Psychoanalytic Institute on a once- or twice-weekly basis over a four- to six-month-period. The department's sole interest was in the validity of the project as a training device. An evaluation of the participants was not intended or carried out.

Prior to the initial meeting of the residents with their preceptors, there was a good deal of discussion as to what the project would entail. Some residents anticipated a miniature analysis geared to familiarizing students with principles of psychoanalysis (i.e., learning by doing). Others felt the project would take a more didactic bent;

> I expected it to be a kind of didactic experience, hoping on one hand it would be a good teaching experience, that I would learn something about something specific, some body of knowledge, or some terminology.

Whether the participants in the project expected a primarily didactic or therapeutic encounter, however, all were certain that they would shortly be involved in

> exploring one thing or another about myself, whether it was something that I or a patient did in therapy, or exploring some more personal or individual kinds of feelings, or exploring my thinking about ideas and about therapy.

Once begun, the project came to be viewed variously as "a psychological tutorial," "a personalized learning experience," or an "intimate experience with psychoanalytic therapy."

Although the residents' expectations were not entirely congruent with the project's reality, they provided an extremely useful set in that each resident came prepared to share his feelings and experiences with someone whom he felt would be receptive and responsive. The set and the reality combined to create what one resident regarded as a valuable learning experience, a period in which thoughts about oneself in relation to the profession were clarified, and an opportunity to formulate and reconcile doubts and feelings concerning the value of psychotherapy for both the resident and the patient.

Three types of learning can be identified as characteristic of the project: intellectual, experiential, and apperceptive. Intellectual learning involves a process that primarily makes use of reasoned inference and abstract thought. Through discussing theoretical and practical issues, the preceptor attempts to enhance the student's knowledge about psychological matters. His appeal is to the intellect and he assumes an essentially professorial role. Drawing upon an established body of knowledge, the preceptor works on sharpening the resident's capacity to develop and deal with psychological concepts. Experiential learning differs from intellectual learning in that subjective experience is used as the base from which knowledge is derived. Perhaps Ford (1963) has stated the argument favoring such learning most succinctly: "Theoretic concepts of the mind and its functions do not become part of the means of psychotherapy until they have been meaningfully experienced on a subjective emotional level." The process of experiential learning begins with the presentation of subjective data. This material is then translated to theoretic constructs through labeling. The construct, its derivation, and its relation to the extant body of psychological knowledge are then explored on a more abstract level.

For example, one resident came away from a meeting feeling that the preceptor had been extremely critical. That afternoon, while participating in a case conference, he engaged the chief of service in an argument and denounced him angrily. The following week the resident related the experience to the analyst. He remarked that he had been angered by the preceptor's criticism. The preceptor then raised the question as to whether the resident's behavior toward his chief was in any way related to what had transpired during their last meeting. During the discussion that followed the resident scrutinized his behavior with the chief of service and concluded that he was treating the chief in the same way he felt the preceptor had treated him. This behavior was then labeled as an example of displacement and identification with the aggressor. The resident and preceptor then went on to talk about the historical background of the concepts and the pertinent literature. Thus, labeling serves as an intermediate step which precedes reasoned inference or abstract thought. Personal experience, behaviors, and feelings are the raw material that, when presented by the student, are then identified by the preceptor as examples of psychological phenomena which can be categorized.

The residents felt labeling altered the abstract quality of theory by introducing a new, more concrete dimension of subjective experience. In the process, the luxury of isolating and intellectualizing affective experiences was removed, and at the same time analytic theory was stripped of some of its mystery:

> When I used words like resistance, transference, they were abstractions. I became acutely aware of the feelings associated with these terms, and as a result, many of the concepts, techniques, and terms which had previously been vague became clear, and a lot of the mystical and/or magical thinking surrounding psychoanalysis was dispelled.

Apperceptive learning represents the third type of learning characteristic of the project. Here, knowledge is derived directly from concrete experience; the preceptor does not serve as an intermediary. Apperceptive learning, exemplified by those situations where patienthood and project coincided, was facilitated by the fact that the participants never fully relinquished their initial fantasy that the project would take the form of a "miniature analysis." Waiting in the analyst's office, they reported a heightened awareness of their own feelings concerning coming to an appointment on time, and frequently found themselves ruminating about what they would say and what they wanted to avoid. For example, one resident said,

> There it was, a mock therapy that allowed you to put yourself into the patient's shoes and to feel what it was like to wait in the waiting room, to go in and sit down, to have to talk, and look forward to 50 minutes of talking, and then to look forward to seven days of thinking over what was said.

Another resident offered,

> Suddenly you're really a patient. You're going to a doctor's office and sitting in the waiting room. There's a secretary typing and you wonder if she is going to send you a bill. This really added significantly to the identity of yourself as a patient.

The participants felt the "as-if" experience of the preceptorship enhanced their appreciation of the dilemmas associated with the patient role. This was brought home most forcefully at the project's end, which coincided with the end of the first year of residency. Residents found themselves exploring their feelings toward the preceptor, reflecting on the difficulties encountered during the meetings, and evaluating how the project had altered their first year of residency. Some experienced termination as denial, others were surprised at how hard it was to say good-bye, and still others found themselves becoming angry and belligerent. All were able to relate these feelings to similar experiences that they were having concurrently with their patients.

Fleckles (1972), in describing his own fellow residents' experiences, suggests that the identity crisis of the first year is mainly resolved by turning to peers and supervisors. The crucial factor for him seemed to be the supervisor's willingness and ability to act as a role model by openly sharing attitudes about psychiatry and allowing the resident to discuss his professional concerns and so develop self-awareness. In the project, one of the major functions of the preceptor was clearly as a role model.

By providing the resident with an opportunity to discuss the problems he is experiencing in becoming a psychiatrist with an established practitioner, the project facilitated the consolidation of a new professional identity and eased the transition into residency. A resident explained, "The edge is off my anxiety about doing psychotherapy and my professional identity seems more solidified as the result of talking to another psychiatrist about what it is to be a psychiatrist."

Although the goals of the project were far too cricumscribed to be considered formal psychotherapy, there is evidence to suggest that the experience was a form of psychotherapy, though it was not being called such by virtue of an implicit "gentlemen's agreement" between participants.

Conceptually, the project stands somewhat between traditional supervision and psychotherapy and contains elements of both pure instruction and therapeutic relief. The preceptorship provides a didactic-therapeutic framework that enables residents to explore professional and personal experiences in such a way as to contribute materially to their theoretical knowledge and technical acumen. It should be viewed as a potential training adjunct that facilitates the learning of psychodynamic constructs while assisting trainees in negotiating the transition into residency.

The Emerging Mentor

But the mentee does not only engage the mentor. The reverse is equally true. And just as the therapist does not emerge fully formed from the psychotherapeutic process, neither does the supervisor. Becoming a supervisor is every bit as much of a developmental experience as becoming a therapist. As mentioned earlier in this chapter, the process of becoming a supervisor begins with the first experience as a supervisee and continues throughout the training years.

In order to focus more clearly on the supervisor and his development, let us first consider the student in transition, the process of disengagement from this training experience. Silberger (1969) writes:

> As a step in the development of professional integration a young psychiatrist after finishing his residency will be noted to pour his energy into a process of active mourning over the loss of his training experience, his colleagues, his patients, his old habit of thought. He struggles with the need to defend the orthodoxy of his past from the challenges of new situations, composing sober, perhaps maudlin or even outraged evaluations of what he has learned and where he has been short-changed in his training. Gradually he can look at the old place with new eyes, deploring or applauding the inevitable changes and feeling the differences within himself as he gives himself the time and the clinical opportunity to grow new objectives and

new perspectives. This mourning process occurs whether he goes away or
stays close to home and seems to depend more on internal needs than on
external circumstances. (p. 108)

We would describe those internal needs as part of the process of
narcissistic (1) engagement, (2) absorption, and (3) dissolution and
mourning, which take place in relation to mentors and institutions in
the service of the development of an adult work identity.

Once the role as student is *formally* ended, the role of supervisor
may *formally* begin. As described above, the transition from one to the
other is not simple, does not occur in a moment, and is just as much in
the service of development as becoming a student.

The Gratification of Supervising

We might ask the question why one becomes a teacher and supervisor. Silberger listed several reasons which we would classify as powerful developmental needs. They are (1) a forum for the exchange of
ideas; (2) friends; (3) narcissistic gratification of trainees and peers; (4) a
framework in which to continue to elaborate professional identity; (5) a
place for ventilation and displacement of affects from patients; and (6)
power and prestige through academic position which may include academic rank, selection of candidates, and supervision.

Focusing more specifically on the supervisor's role, it is clear that
one supervises to meet multiple, powerful developmental needs. In his
role as mentor, the supervisor has a need to see his student learn, progress, and develop. But there are contrasting internal demands other
than those just described. Wishes to be admired, aggrandized, and imi-
tated—the reasons the sorcerer has an apprentice—are powerful forces
within the supervisor. Competitive feelings are also present which
may, if not recognized, result in attempts to impede student growth.
Finally, supervising fulfills an important developmental need of caring
for and facilitating the young—a direct application of Erikson's idea of
generativity. By involving himself, the midlife adult experiences a
sense of continuity with his own adult past and with the future of his
profession through his involvement with mentees.

In many academic situations, particularly postgraduate master's
and doctoral programs, the mentor/advisor/supervisor has enormous
power over his students and may literally control their lives, particularly in relation to the doctoral dissertation. Unless the middle-aged or

older mentor is aware of and controls feelings of jealousy and envy of his student's youth, sexuality, and creativity, the potential for great abuse of this power exists. *Recognition* of the narcissistic issues in the mentee–mentor relationship and the developmental needs of *both* student and teacher may allow the relationship to be mutually beneficial.

A clear example of the way in which supervisory situations are abused is in the relationship between male academic supervisors and female doctoral students. On occasion these situations have developed into ones of sexual exploitation. Consciously or unconsciously the mentor knows that his student is in a vulnerable, dependent position. If the student does not submit to sexual advances, she fears educational retaliation. This kind of exploitation is a particularly important problem in the career development of women because of the relative absence of female mentors and the cultural acceptance of female sexual exploitation.

The Use of Developmental Concepts in Supervision

The developmental orientation provides the supervisor with concepts that clarify the goals of supervision. According to Ornstein (1968) the basic skills of the future therapist reach a certain level of development in his own experiences prior to training. In supervision "our pedagogic task is to render these basic skills of the trainee available for *further development*, to broaden, deepen, and sharpen them" (p. 298, italics added).

This recognition that the therapist is in the midst of a developmental process that specifically deals with the establishment of his professional identity is important because it *organizes* the supervisor's interaction with the therapist. According to Martin and Prosen (1976), the supervisor should help the new therapist recognize that "his concerns about his competence and identity are not indications of his unsuitability for psychotherapy nor are they sure indications of neurotic conflict" (p. 132). This simple recognition allows the therapist to more accurately attune his own reactions in the ongoing therapeutic process.

We agree with Gutmann (1971) that it is the supervisor's task to undermine the prevalent assumption concerning middle and later life that

> true psychological development ends with physical maturation, and that the individual coasts through the rest of his life acting out the traumas and

acting on the capacities that are the residues of the early developmental years" (p. 237).

If that basic assumption is prevalent in the mind of the beginning (or experienced) therapist, it will determine how he weighs what the patient says and what *he* says to the patient, slanting techniques toward genetic material and away from material related to adaptation in the current reality.

In illustrating this concept, Martin and Prosen (1976) speak of its usefulness in understanding the meaning of regression. "Regression, which takes its meaning by its contrast with age-appropriate behavior, can only be clearly conceptualized if there is an articulate understanding of what is age appropriate" (p. 128). With adult patients this "articulate understanding" must be based on a knowledge of adult development.

Supervision must center around such developmental issues as *age* and *phase differences* between patient and therapist. Martin and Prosen give the example of a woman in her fifties and a therapist in his late twenties, only several years older than the patient's children. The patient complains that the therapist is too young to understand her. This is a common complaint in training interactions, which usually causes the beginning therapist considerable anxiety. The threatened therapist may respond in several ways: (1) He may attempt to act like the wise sage, a position open to criticism by the patient because of his youth and inexperience. (2) To protect himself, he may assume that the patient is really talking about infantile issues. This belief is comforting and compensatory since *both* therapist and patient have grown beyond those levels. Furthermore, the stance gives the therapist an additional edge because he knows, theoretically, what happened in childhood while the patient may not. (3) He may attempt to diminish the age difference by revealing his own adult experiences, or calling the patient by her first name.

There are, of course, other examples of the effect of age and developmental difference on therapy. For instance, the therapist may try to obliterate the age difference between himself and an adolescent patient, "hoping to secure the patient's trust and to avoid indiscriminate anger turned toward the adult world" (Martin & Prosen, 1976, p. 131). Or an older therapist may see all patients—or students, we would add—as needing a warm, wise parent.

Another example of our own focuses on a case, presented in supervision by an experienced therapist, of a woman in her fifties.

> Recently divorced, she had moved away from her former husband and children to take a job opportunity. The supervisee failed to conceptualize what it meant to be 50 and focused instead on the history of deprivation in childhood and on the dynamics of her depression. Was chemotherapy indicated? he asked. As relevant as those questions were, they failed to focus on the patient's loneliness, mourning for her marriage, and apprehension about getting old alone because of earlier neglect of her children. The therapist was encouraged to engage her around those issues *first* in order to build a therapeutic alliance and avoid the loss of the patient, already hinted at by her after a few visits.

The Supervisory Triangle

The developmental orientation provides additional insight into the supervisory process when it is recognized that the interaction occurring in supervision is the result of what we call the "supervisory triangle." That triangle consists of the patient, the therapist, and the supervisor. Not only are three individuals involved, but three *developing* individuals.

The triangle is *unique* in each instance because the ages, developmental levels, and current circumstances of the individuals involved are always different and in flux.

Implicit in this concept is the recognition that what transpires in supervision is determined by all three of the individuals involved although only two are actually present. *Both* supervisor and supervisee react to the patient in terms of their own past and current experience. For example, the therapist in his late twenties may not be as attuned to a late adolescent as the supervisor who has a child of that age. Therapist and supervisor react to each other in an infinite variety of ways determined by their conscious and unconscious attitudes toward each other and their positions in the life cycle.

It is incumbent on the supervisor to be cognizant of both his own and the supervisee's position in the life cycle and to be aware of how both of them are handling the developmental tasks in their lives. The specifics of their interaction with each other and with the patient will be clarified by such an approach.

Demonstration Courses, Student Reports, and Comments

In the final section of this chapter we shall present two demonstration courses illustrating the use of child- and adult-developmental concepts. The first, entitled "The Psychoanalytic Theory of Adult Development," is given by us biannually at the San Diego Psychoanalytic Institute; the second, "The Developmental Case Conference," is offered annually to first-year adult psychiatric residents at the University of California at San Diego.

The Normal Development of Adulthood

"The Psychoanalytic Theory of Adult Development" is a 12-seminar (2 hours) course for third- and fourth-year analytic candidates. The purpose of the seminars is to integrate data on normal adulthood from biological, sociological, and psychological spheres with existing psychodynamic theory and clinical experience, leading toward a comprehensive psychoanalytic theory of adulthood. Although presented to psychoanalytic candidates, much of the material is suitable for students of other disciplines at the graduate level and some at the undergraduate level. It is our hope that these basic articles will be studied and elaborated on by all students of human behavior.

SEMINAR I: An Overview: Developmental Psychology and the Life Cycle

1. Gould, R. L. The phases of adult life: A study in developmental psychology. *American Journal of Psychiatry,* 1973, *129,* 521–531.
2. Levinson, D. The psychosocial development of men in early adulthood and the midlife transition. *Life History Research in Psychopathology, 3,* 1974, 243–258.
3. Roazen, P. The life cycle. In E. H. Erikson (Ed.), *The power and limits of a vision.* New York: Free Press, 1976, pp. 107–120.
4. Conference on Psychoanalytic Education and Research. Commission IX, "Child Analysis." New York: American Psychoanalytic Association, 1974, pp. 1–20.

GOAL: To introduce basic developmental concepts on adulthood.

SEMINAR II: The Frontier: Some Basic Observations and Hypotheses about Adult Development

1. Colarusso, C. A., & Nemiroff, R. A. Some observations and hypotheses about the psychoanalytic theory of adult development. *International Journal of Psycho-Analysis*, 1979, *60*, 59–72.

GOAL: *To present the basic questions in the field of adult development which need exploration and elaboration.*

SEMINAR III. Separation–Individuation throughout the Life Cycle

1. Winestine, M. (Reporter). The experience of separation–individuation in infancy and its reverberations through the course of life: Infancy and childhood (Panel report). *Journal of the American Psychoanalytic Association*, 1973, *21*, 135–154.
2. Marcus, I. (Reporter). The experience of separation–individuation in infancy and its reverberations through the course of life: Adolescence and maturity (Panel report). *Journal of the American Psychoanalytic Association*, 1973, *21*, 155–167.
3. Steinschein, I. (Reporter). The experience of separation–individuation in infancy and its reverberations through the course of life: Maturity, senescence, and sociological implications (Panel report). *Journal of the American Psychoanalytic Association*, 1973, *21*, 633–645.

GOAL: *To present one of the very few important theoretical constructs that has been conceptualized developmentally throughout the life cycle.*

SEMINAR IV: The Development of the Mind in Adulthood

1. Pribram, K. *Languages of the brain: Experimental paradoxes and principles in neuropsychology.* Englewood Cliffs, N.J.: Prentice-Hall, 1971, pp. 27–47.
2. Vaillant, G. *Adaptation to life.* Boston: Little, Brown, 1977, pp. 329–350.
3. Kimmel, D. *Adulthood and aging: An interdisciplinary developmental view.* New York: Wiley, 1976, pp. 276–390.

GOAL: *To explore the idea that the mind and its biological substrate, the brain, continue to evolve in adulthood.*

SEMINAR V: The Development of Psychic Structure in Adulthood:
The Adult Self

1. Saperstein, J. L., & Gaines, J. Metapsychological considerations
   of the self. *International Journal of Psycho-Analysis*, 1973, *54*,
   415–423.
2. Nemiroff, R. A., & Colarusso, C. A. Authenticity and narcissism in the adult development of the self. *The Annual of Psychoanalysis*, 1980, *8*.
3. Rangell, L. The role of the parent in the Oedipus complex. *Bulletin of the Menninger Clinic*, 1955, *19*, 9–15.
4. Colarusso, C. A., & Nemiroff, R. A. The father at midlife: Crisis
   and growth of paternal identity. In S. Cath, A. Gurwitt, & J. M.
   Ross (Eds.), *Fatherhood*. Boston: Little, Brown, in press.

*GOAL: To describe the adult evolution of one form of psychic structure, the
self; and to illustrate, through parenthood, how that happens.*

SEMINAR VI: The Adult Developmental Aspects of Love and Intimacy

1. Kernberg, O. Mature love: Prerequisites and characteristics.
   Journal of the American Psychoanalytic Association, 1974, *22*,
   743–768.
2. Binstock, W. Two forms of intimacy. *Journal of the American Psychoanalytic Association*, 1973, *21*, 93–108.
3. Lidz, T. *The person: His development throughout the life cycle*. New
   York: Basic Books, 1968, pp. 410–439.
4. Erikson, E. H. *Childhood and society*. New York: W. W. Norton,
   1963, pp. 263–268.

*GOAL: To consider the developmental aspects of the major adult experiences of
intimacy, love, and marriage.*

SEMINAR VII: The Adult-Developmental Aspects of Pregnancy and
Parenthood

1. Bibring, G., Dwyer, T. F., Huntington, D. S., & Valenstein,
   A. F. A study of the psychological processes in pregnancy and
   the earliest mother-child relationship. *Psychoanalytic Study of the
   Child*, 1961, *16*, 9–26.
2. Benedek, T. *Parenthood: Its psychology and psychopathology*. Boston: Little, Brown, 1970, pp. 285–306.

3. Parents, H. (Reporter). Parenthood as a developmental phase (Panel report). *Journal of the American Psychoanalytic Association,* 1975, *23,* 154–165.

GOAL: *To explore the developmental aspects of the major adult experiences of pregnancy and parenthood.*

SEMINAR VIII: Work and Play in Adulthood

1. Freud, Anna. The Concept of Developmental Lines (The line from the body to the toy and from play to work). *Psychoanalytic Study of the Child,* 1963, *18,* 258–262.
2. Szasz, Thomas S. The Experience of the Analyst. *Journal of the American Psychoanalytic Association,* 1956, *4,* 197–223.
3. Adatto, Carl. On Play and the Psychopathology of Golf. *Journal of the American Psychoanalytic Association,* 1965, *12,* 826–841.
4. Drellich, Marvin. The Interrelationships of Work and Play. In J. H. Masserman (Ed.), *The dynamics of work and marriage (Science and psychoanalysis,* Vol. 16). New York: Grune & Stratton, 1970, pp. 17–26.

GOAL: *To explore the nature of work and play in adulthood.*

SEMINAR IX: Time Sense throughout the Life Cycle

1. Colarusso, C. A. The development of time sense: From birth to object constancy. *International Journal of Psycho-Analysis,* 1979, *60,* 242–252.
2. Seaton, P. The psycho-temporal adaptation of late adolescence. *Journal of the American Psychoanalytic Association,* 1974, *22,* 795–819.
3. Kafka, J. S. (Reporter). The experience of time (Panel report). *Journal of the American Psychoanalytic Association,* 1972, *20,* 650–657.
4. Bonaparte, M. Time and the unconscious. *International Journal of Psycho-Analysis,* 1940, *21,* 427–468.

GOAL: *To study the subjective nature of time sense and its changing perception and effect on development at different developmental phases.*

SEMINAR X: Death: A Developmental Stimulus to Health

    1. Freud, S. *Thoughts for the times on war and death.* Standard edition, 14: 289–300. London: Hogarth Press, 1915.
    2. Jacques, E. Death and the mid-life crisis. *International Journal of Psycho-Analysis,* 1965, 46, 502–514.

GOAL: To explore the central preoccupation with death at midlife and explore its effects from a developmental standpoint.

SEMINAR XI: Clinical Applications of Developmental Theory

    1. Shane, M. A rationale for teaching analytic technique based on a developmental orientation and approach. *International Journal of Psycho-Analysis,* 1977, 58, 95–108.
    2. Ornstein, P. H. Sorcerer's apprentice: The initial phase of training and education in psychiatry. *Comprehensive Psychiatry,* 1968, 9, 293–315.
    3. Clinical presentations from seminar members.

GOALS: To present some basic ideas on the application of developmental concepts to teaching and training and to hear clinical presentations from seminar members illustrating their grasp of developmental concepts. An example is presented at the end of this seminar outline.

SEMINAR XII: Clinical Applications of Developmental Theory (continued)

    1. Shane, M. The developmental approach to "working through" in the analytic process. *International Journal of Psycho-Analysis,* 1979, 60, 375–382.
    2. Martin, R. M., & Prosen, H. Psychotherapy, supervision, and life tasks. *Bulletin of the Menninger Clinic,* 1976, 40, 125–133.
    3. Prosen, H., & Martin, R. M. The developmental point of view and its implications for psychotherapy. *The Psychiatric Journal of the University of Ottawa,* 1978, 3, 183–188.
    4. Clinical presentations from seminar members.

GOALS: To explore the relationship between developmental concepts and psychotherapy and psychoanalysis and to hear clinical presentations from seminar members.

Sample Clinical Presentations

In the last two seminars of the course, students were asked to present clinical material illustrating the use of the developmental concepts described in the course. The examples show how new insights into the experience of marriage and parenthood affected the therapists' work with their patients.

Sample I. Adult Development: Clinical Vignettes of Psychological Growth from the Experience of Parenting

Situation. A 39-year-old obsessional male in analysis because of complaints of marital dissatisfaction presents evidence of shifting behavior and fantasies toward his 5-, 11-, and 13-year-old daughters.

Developmental Phase of Adulthood. Early and middle parenting, as conceptualized by Therese Benedek.

Developmental Tasks. Individuation of self and modulation of instinctual life with new defensive/adaptive structures precipitated by interactions with his children. Adaptive shifts complicated by normal unconscious identification with children (and "family" setting) leading to a reactivation of parent conflicts from childhood and adolescence.

Parenting Realities and Corresponding Behavior Presented Initially in Analysis. 1. Birth of first child: "She became a mother . . . had no time for me . . . I felt now everyone knew that I had been screwing . . . I guess I felt that I had to be a good boy and couldn't play . . . maybe that is why I started staying away and having affairs."

2. Birth of second child: "Hell, I'm a second child and turned out all right . . . why should she have her own bedroom just because her older sister does . . . I had to learn that the world isn't fair."

3. Birth of third child: "Aren't I man enough to have a son . . . I wish she would go away . . . she cried because I threw her in the can with the grass cuttings. If she were a boy I could teach her to mow it . . . I keep dreaming of Joe, the six-year-old son of this girl I'm hustling at work . . . I encouraged her to go hunting with me, but maybe I shouldn't have bought her such a big gun, the kick knocks her down."

4. Sexuality of oedipal and pubescent daughters: "No, there aren't any sexual feelings . . . with your own kids . . . why not walk around nude and take showers together, it's not as if I got an erection . . . the

little one is always pestering me, trying to get on my lap . . . I have to close the door just to take a piss . . . I couldn't get it on in this dream because these little girls were peeking over the bed."

5. Dependency of children: "I really smacked her when she started crying over her skinned knee . . . I can't stand their whimpering . . . it's always 'buy this, buy that' but they'll never set the table."

Parenting Realities and Corresponding Behavior One Year Later. 1. Growing empathic awareness of children's sexuality: "I guess at 13 my daughter has to be a little shy around me . . . not the little one though, she is the sexiest of the lot . . . I keep telling the 11-year-old her boobs will grow in good time; I told her how upset I was as an underdeveloped adolescent."

2. Growing acceptance of childhood dependency and fears of helplessness and inadequacy: "The middle one keeps thinking I won't love her if she doesn't get all A's . . . I told her she is her own worst critic."

3. Separation in inner world of mother-of-self from mother-of-children (partial): "I don't want to sleep with anyone else . . . I don't love her as I once did, but at least it is sex . . . I can see how hard those kids are to handle all day."

4. A general emergence, expression, and resolution of adolescent ambitions: "My mother wouldn't let me buy a motorcycle, but no one can stop me now . . . although I'll probably sell it down the line when I see guys getting hurt . . . it's as if I have to relive my adolescence a bit."

5. An expanding awareness of his emotional realities as a child, including sibling rivalry, sibling sexuality, dependent and libidinal strivings toward parents (a continuing dynamic development of the oedipal complex as conceptualized by Rangell).

Presumed Determinants of Behavioral Shifts. Pressures for adaptive behavior at home. Analytic work within a positive parental transference with a major focus on confronting denial in areas of parental ambitions.

Inferred Structural Shifts. A lifting of repression allowing for an appreciation of and permissiveness toward child and adolescent sexuality. Behavioral examination leading to an awareness of parent introjects which may then be reintegrated in a less prohibitive, restrictive fashion. Shift to a less primitive superego and a less grandiose ego ideal, allowing for greater pride. Children viewed as more separate, and thus greater room for empathy allowed.

Major Shifts in Defensive Mechanisms. The patient's initial behaviors were marked by denial, projection, global identifications, acting out, and repetitive compulsion. Recent behavior indicates a greater capacity for suppression, altruism (empathy), and humor. Gradual clearing of the pathological investments in children has allowed for a greater capacity for investment in his wife, work, and analysis.

Sample II: Case History

A 44-year-old, married mother of three children L., was referred by her daughter because of outbursts of unprovoked anger, depression, and suicidal ideation. The patient had successfully raised three children, now grown, and the youngest, a son, was involved in what was for him a very difficult, painful process of leaving home. From the time her children became adolescents, L. had gone back to work, where she functioned well. She had had two previous episodes of psychiatric treatment for depression and was once hospitalized briefly. Her tendency to become withdrawn and depressed from time to time was burdensome to her husband, but much more so at this time than ever before.

She herself was the last born of three children. Her mother hoped for a boy and didn't warm up to her daughter until well into the second year of life. During this time her much older sister and father provided most the care. The father read to her and instilled in her a quest for learning. The patient grew up trying to please her mother by competing with men in school. She had the hope that she herself would go to medical school, perhaps in this way fulfilling her mother's expectations of a son. She was academically successful and got scholarships, but her educational goals stopped after getting her Master's degree because she worked to put her older brother through graduate school and she met, fell in love with, and married her husband.

The patient's husband worked successfully in an upper management position. Although he had tried to be understanding of his wife's gradual emotional withdrawal into sleeping, housework, and self-pity, he hoped she would work herself out of it. But he and the children finally lost patience and insisted she go for help. He put it simply if not boldly: "The kids are grown and have their own lives and that doesn't mean I don't want to continue to be helpful to them, but now I need her and she just isn't there. I want her to be there for us now, we've gone through a lot together, but if she can't be a wife and a friend to me, and if you can't help her with this either, I'll have to leave her and try to find someone else who can."

I was startled by his candor and his telling me exactly what I also thought had to occur for there to be a successful resolution to this problem. My patient had to reestablish her relationship with her husband.

Despite some difficult periods, it has been adequate and gratifying for many years previously. She now had to allow herself to be needed and valued primarily as spouse as opposed to mother, a process which was fraught with danger to this woman's self-esteem because as a parent she could restitutively compensate for inadequacies of the parenting she received.

The diagnosis was neurotic depression, severe, and the treatment was twice-weekly psychotherapy. The early part of the treatment focused on the many genetic determinants of the present problems. But we soon became involved in searching for ways to get back into the track of development, which meant (1) analyzing obstacles in the way of her gradually giving up her excessive attachment to the children (for instance, she would not give away or throw out their old clothes so their rooms could be repainted), and (2) becoming more involved with her husband (for instance, she avoided getting together with old friends, couples). It soon became clear to me that we could not indefinitely analyze the genetic basis to the obstacles to her further development, because life goes on, either with her or without her; just as the school-age child cannot indefinitely put off going to school, and the adolescent cannot completely avoid considerations of sex and dating, she had to take some steps in order to continue her development, or risk losing her husband.

This was evidently a time of considerable stress in their marriage and the marriage was obviously very important to her future. It was necessary for me to do what I could to help her preserve it. Clinically this meant that it was necessary to actively focus on such seemingly mundane matters as what interfered with their plans to "double date" with another couple. This therapeutic path had certain pitfalls since it seemed to her at times that I was siding with her husband rather than with her development. A here-and-now approach to the specific difficulties in her relationship to her husband, facilitating her mourning the loss of the children and remaking an attachment to her husband, was helpful at this point.

Eventually she became less withdrawn and more emotionally available to her husband. She also showed much change in several severe physical problems; her allergies diminished considerably so she could return to the yard work, which she loved, and her irritable-bowel syndrome, with its sometimes debilitating diarrhea, quieted down. She started to clean out the children's old clothes and went out with her husband and other couples. Sexually she became more interested in her husband and helped him with his premature ejaculation.

All this allowed her husband to take advantage of a promotion that meant a move to another city. She found that it was difficult to rent the house and leave the city where her children had grown up, but she managed it skillfully. Our work was not finished, and we both knew she still needed some assistance to finish what we started, so I helped her to locate a new therapist in the city to which she moved. The last that I heard, she was doing well.

The Developmental Case Conference: An Introductory Course for First-Year Psychiatric Residents

In an attempt to *introduce* the developmental orientation to psychiatric residents, the authors devised and taught a course that introduced theoretical and clinical concepts illustrated by case presentations. The course was followed in the second and third years of training, using the spiral curriculum concept, by further lectures, case presentations, and clinical exposure to children and adults. The course is designed to integrate clinical and theoretical material and actively involves the beginning residents and the more advanced child fellows as presenters and teachers, thus facilitating the development of their own professional identities.

The goals of this series are the following: (1) The concepts of normal child and adult development will be presented; (2) case material from both inpatient wards and the child-guidance clinic will be coordinated with the developmental concepts; and (3) specific psychodynamic concepts useful in diagnostic and therapeutic work will be presented in conjunction with case material.

Schedule of Conference Topics

1. "Taking a Developmental Case History": An outline of how to take a developmental history will be presented to the residents, as well as a specific sample of a developmental case history.

2. "Case Conference": A first-year resident will present a case illustrating the use of the developmental history in a diagnosis and treatment plan.

3. "Normal Development I": Psychodynamic theory covering the first six years of life, illustrated with clinical examples—a lecture.

4. "Case Conference": A child case illustrating normal and pathological development in the first six years of life will be presented by a Child Fellow.

5. "Normal Development II': Psychodynamic theory covering latency and adolescence, illustrated with clinical examples—a lecture.

6. "Case Conference": A case illustrating normal and pathological development in adolescence will be presented by a Child Fellow.

7. "Basic Developmental Dynamics": Concepts relating to diagnosis and treatment such as regression, fixation, and working through will be presented with case illustrations—a lecture.

8. "Normal Development III": Psychodynamic theory covering the young-adult years, illustrated with clinical examples—a lecture.

9. "Case Conference": A case presentation, illustrating normal and pathological aspects of early-adult development, will be presented by a first-year resident.

10. "Normal Development IV": Psychodynamic theory covering middle and old age, illustrated with clinical examples—a lecture.

11. "Case Conference": A case presentation illustrating normal and pathological aspects of late-adult development will be presented by a first-year resident.

REFERENCES

Conference on Psychoanalytic Education and Research. Commission IX, "Child Analysis." New York: American Psychoanalytic Association, 1974.

Fleckles, A. The making of a psychiatrist: The resident's view of the process of his professional development. *American Journal of Psychiatry*, 1972, *128*, 101.

Ford, E. S. D. Being and becoming a psychotherapist. *American Journal of Psychotherapy*, 1963, *27*, 472.

Gutmann, D. Cross-cultural research on human behavior: A comparative study of the life cycle in the middle and later years. In N. Kretchmer & D. Walcher (Eds.), *Environmental influences and genetic expression*. Fogarty International Center Proceedings, No. 2. Washington, D.C.: United States Government Printing Office, 1971, p. 237.

Martin, R. M., & Prosen, H. Psychotherapy, supervision and life tasks: The younger therapist and the middle-aged patient. *Bulletin of the Menninger Clinic*, 1976, *40*, 125.

Nemiroff, R. A., & Tischler, G. L. A preceptorship for beginning psychiatric residents. *Journal of Psychiatric Education*, 1977, *1*, 167.

Ornstein, P. Sorcerer's apprentice: Training and education in psychiatry. *Comprehensive Psychiatry*, 1968, *9*, 293.

Ritvo, S. Psychoanalysis as science and profession: Prospects and changes. *Journal of the American Psychoanalytic Association*, 1971, *19*, 3.

Silberger, J. The supervisor's rewards. In E. Semrad & D. Van Buskirk (Eds.), *Teaching psychotherapy of psychotic patients*. New York: Grune & Stratton, 1964, pp. 106–115.

Van Buskirk, D. Identity development in the beginning psychiatrist. In E. Semrad & D. Van Buskirk (Eds.), *Teaching psychotherapy of psychotic patients*. New York: Grune & Stratton, 1969, pp. 45–64.

Index

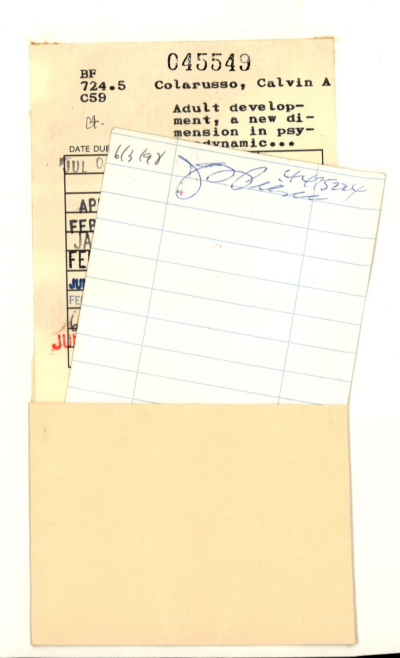